E-Cigarette Smoking, Voice, and Health

Abdul-latif Hamdan

E-Cigarette Smoking, Voice, and Health

A Clinician's Guide to Vaping's Effect on Voice and Breathing

Springer

Abdul-latif Hamdan
Department of Otolaryngology - Head and Neck Surgery
American University of Beirut Medical Center
Beirut, Lebanon

ISBN 978-3-032-04912-4 ISBN 978-3-032-04913-1 (eBook)
https://doi.org/10.1007/978-3-032-04913-1

This Springer imprint is published by the registered company Springer Nature Switzerland AG
The registered company address is: Gewerbestrasse 11, 6330 Cham, Switzerland

This book is dedicated to my wife Sawsan for her constant love and support and to my children, Aya, Adam, and Jad, for being the light of my life.

Preface

Electronic cigarettes represent a distinct type of nicotine delivery system that relies on heat rather than combustion to convert a solvent into an aerosol. The number of ever-e-cigarette users and current users in the United States and around the globe has markedly increased over the years, mostly over the last decade. The surge in the use of e-cigarettes among adolescents is even higher than that reported in adults. One of the reasons is that e-cigarettes are advertised as a safer alternative to combustion cigarettes. Numerous reports in the literature indicate that a large percentage of cigarette smokers have started using e-cigarettes with the belief that it is less harmful than traditional cigarettes, and that vaping would help them stop or at least reduce smoking. Nonetheless, there is increasing evidence that e-cigarette use also has adverse effects on health, leading to a constellation of symptoms.

E-Cigarette Smoking, Voice, and Health: A Clinician's Guide to Vaping's Effect on Voice and Breathing provides an overview on the impact of e-cigarette use on various systems in the body, with an emphasis on voice. Chapter 1 reviews the prevalence of e-cigarette use globally and the associated intents and beliefs among vapors. Chapter 2 summarizes the impact of e-cigarette use on health, with an emphasis on the ear, nose, and throat. Chapters 3–5 offer background information on the clinical anatomy and physiology of phonation, the work-up of a patient with voice disorders, and insights on the most common vocal fold pathologies encountered in otolaryngology practice. Chapter 6 highlights the voice symptoms in e-cigarette users, while Chap. 7 directs the reader toward the adverse effect of vaping on the power source of phonation, namely breathing. The increased risk of infection and bronchial epithelia dysfunction in smokers are discussed. Chapters 8 examines the link between vaping and diseases of the oral cavity, and Chap. 9 discusses the effect of vaping on nose and paranasal sinus diseases, with an emphasis on ciliary beating dysfunction in smokers. Chapter 10 highlights smoking in general as a risk factor for reflux disease and the etiologic role of this latter in patients with voice disorders.

E-Cigarette Smoking, Voice, and Health: A Clinician's Guide to Vaping's Effect on Voice and Breathing summarizes the current reports in the literature on the impact of e-cigarette use on voice and health. The content of this manuscript can help provide a platform for future research on vaping, voice, and systemic diseases.

Beirut, Lebanon

Abdul-latif Hamdan

Acknowledgment

Sincere acknowledgment and thanks to Dr. Lana Ghzayel for her thorough assistance in formatting the manuscript and editing the references for publication.

Contents

Part I

Introduction

E-Cigarette Smoking: Prevalence, Associated Intents, and Beliefs

1

Electronic cigarettes represent a distinct type of nicotine delivery system that relies on heat rather than combustion to convert a solvent into an aerosol [1]. The basic concept is simple. An e-cigarette is composed of a power source, a heater or atomizing device, and a liquid [2]. The power source, which constitutes the device's largest component, is usually a rechargeable battery. The heater or atomizing device is a coil that gets activated manually or by pressure alteration during inhalation. Lastly, there is a solvent that consists mainly of propylene glycol and glycerol or vegetable glycerin [1, 3]. Other detected compounds include formaldehyde, acetone, ethanol, and others [3]. Nicotine may or may not be present in the solvent, and its concentration varies between various products [2, 4]. Another important addition to the e-liquid is flavorings. This latter has helped spread e-cigarette use across all age groups [5]. Using different flavors in the e-liquid allows e-cigarette smokers to tailor vaping to their liking. By changing the resistance in the heating coil, vapors can also control the density of the aerosol [6, 7].

E-cigarette was first invented in 1963 by Herbert. E. Gilbert as a "smokeless non-tobacco cigarette" [8]. Forty years later, the device was modernized by a Chinese pharmacist named Hon Lik [1, 8]. E-cigarette entered the US market in 2007 [9, 10]. Since its inception, more than 90 companies have been launched, and by 2022 more than 900 e-cigarette brands invaded the market via websites and other online marketing tools [11, 12]. Today, it is estimated that more than 15,000 flavorings are currently available for end users [13]. Different generations of e-cigarettes have evolved over the years. Although the first generation was designed to look like a cigarette, the design has evolved over the years. The second generation, commonly referred to as "vape pens," differed in size, battery power, and e-liquid holding capacity compared to the first generation. The third generation led to an increase in e-cigarette marketing due to its ability to produce denser aerosol, enhancing its appeal among the youth [7]. This was made possible by modifying the heating coil resistance, among other factors. The fourth generation, which looked more like "pod-mods," allowed the end user to change the "pods" [7].

A.-l. Hamdan, *E-Cigarette Smoking, Voice, and Health*,
https://doi.org/10.1007/978-3-032-04913-1_1

Prevalence of E-Cigarette Smoking

The number of ever-e-cigarette users and current users in the United States and around the globe has markedly increased over the years, and mostly over the last decade or so. The surge in the use of e-cigarettes among adolescents is even higher than that reported in adults. In 2013, using a large survey that included 5939 former and current smokers in the United States, Canada, the United Kingdom, and Australia, Akidson et al. reported a higher prevalence of trying electronic nicotine delivery systems (ENDS) among "younger, nondaily high-income smokers" [14]. In 2016, Mirboluk et al. conducted a study on the prevalence and distribution of e-cigarette use among US adults and noted that 4.5% were current users. More than half of these users were below the age of 35 years [15]. In 2017, Wilson et al. used data from a survey that included 34,356 participants and noted that e-cigarette users were younger and poorer than those who never smoked e-cigarettes. The authors also reported a nonlinear relationship between e-cigarette use and education. Participants with college or high school education had higher adjusted odds of ever smoking e-cigarettes [16]. In 2018, Hedman et al. conducted a study looking at the prevalence of smoking among 30,272 randomly selected subjects and found that 9.8% of current smokers (12.3% of the participants) used e-cigarettes. E-cigarette smoking was more common in men, and the odds of using e-cigarettes decreased with age from 2.77 in individuals aged 20–29 years to 1.47 in those aged 50–59 years [17]. In another report on trends in adolescent vaping and the role of e-cigarette smoking in predicting future cigarette smoking, Miech et al. noted that recent vapers who had never smoked a cigarette before were 4 times more likely to report cigarette smoking in the past year. The study was conducted on 347 12th-grade high school students who were randomly selected and resurveyed 1 year later [18]. Similarly, Morean et al. surveyed the use of one type of e-cigarette among students of four different high schools and found that 43.5% were ever or past-month users [19].

In line with the above, the use of e-cigarettes varied with the geographic location and time. In 2018, Yoong et al. conducted a systematic review and meta-analysis on the prevalence of ENDS use among youth globally and noted an increase in their ever use in the United States, Poland, Korea, and New Zealand. The prevalence of ENDS ever use in 2013–2015 was the highest in Poland and the lowest in Italy (62.1% and 5.9%, respectively) [20]. In 2021, in another systematic review with a median sample size of 3925 children and adolescents, the same authors reported a pooled prevalence of 17.2% for ever use of ENDS or electronic non-nicotine delivery system (ENNDS), and 7.8% for their current use [21]. Boakye et al. investigated the patterns in e-cigarette use among adults in the United States and noted an increase in prevalence of current e-cigarette use from 4.4% in 2017 to 5.5% in 2018, and a drop to 5.1% in 2020. Among young adults, there was an increase from 13.5% in 2018 to 14.5% in 2020 [22].

Impact of E-Cigarette Marketing on Vaping

E-cigarette advertisements have expanded over the last decades, leading to an increase in vaping and the use of other smoking products such as cigarettes, hookah, and cigars [23]. Mantey et al. investigated the impact of e-cigarette marketing exposure and found an increase in the likelihood of susceptibility and e-cigarette use as the number of e-cigarette marketing channels increased. There was an association between e-cigarette ever use and current use, and e-cigarette marketing. The study was conducted using the 2014 National Youth Tobacco survey, which included 22,007 middle and high school students [24]. In a sample of 8121 US participants between the ages of 12 and 17 years and 1683 between the ages of 18 and 24 years, Chen-Sankey et al. also reported that exposure to e-cigarette marketing increased the odds of experimenting with e-cigarettes [25]. Cruz et al. conducted a study looking at the impact of marketing exposure on subsequent use of different tobacco products and found that frequent internet and in-store exposure increased the odds of beginning smoking among adolescent never-smokers (OR = 2.98). Moreover, exposure to outdoor e-cigarette marketing and the internet increased the likelihood of initiating e-cigarette use. The authors concluded that there was an association between exposure to marketing tobacco and initiation of smoking [26]. In a survey on the association between online e-cigarette exposure and use among Chinese students, Dai et al. noted that online exposure increased the intention to use e-cigarettes. Almost 74% of their cohort (12,470 participants) knew about e-cigarettes. The main sources of information were the internet, movies, and bulletin boards in 42.4%, 36.4%, and 34.9% of the cases, respectively. Other sources of online information included advertising flyers (33.9%) and friends (13.8%) [27]. Swiatkowska et al. examined the link between e-cigarette advertising and e-cigarette use in 7498 adolescents in Poland. The analysis based on a questionnaire showed that more than half (56%) had been exposed to e-cigarette advertising. Moreover, exposure to e-cigarette advertising increased the odds of ever using e-cigarettes [28]. Last but not least, using group analysis, Smith et al. noted that e-cigarette companies used influencers, among other tactics, to promote the use of their products [29].

E-Cigarette-Associated Intent and Beliefs

E-cigarettes have been advertised as a safer alternative to combustible cigarettes. Based on that premise, numerous reports in the literature indicate that a large percentage of cigarette smokers have started using e-cigarettes with the belief that it is less harmful than traditional cigarettes, and that vaping will help them stop or at least reduce smoking. Although e-cigarettes may or may not contain nicotine in various concentrations, it is thought of by many as a nicotine replacement therapy in addition to other FDA-approved methods such as chewing gum, sucking a lozenge, using a patch, or an inhaler [30]. Etter et al. conducted a survey on 81 ever-users of e-cigarettes and noted that the majority used e-cigarettes to quit or reduce cigarette consumption with the belief that it is less harmful than conventional smoking [31]. In a study on 104 smokers, Foulds et al. noted that three out of four started using e-cigarettes with the intent to stop smoking, and almost two-thirds had previously failed to quit smoking using other FDA-approved smoking cessation medications [32]. In a study on patterns of ENDS awareness and product-associated beliefs of current and former smokers across Canada, the United States, the United Kingdom, and Australia, Akidson et al. noted that 79.8% of the participants believed that ENDS were less harmful than conventional cigarettes. The authors also noted that 75.4% and 85.1% used ENDS to help them reduce or quit smoking, respectively [14]. That same year, in an online survey on e-cigarette use, which included 1347 participants from 33 countries, Dawkins et al. reported an overall impression that e-cigarettes were less harmful and had fewer side effects than traditional smoking. The time for a first cigarette smoke was significantly less than the time for a first vape among ex-smokers [33]. A year later, in a worldwide survey that included 19,414 participants, Farsalinos et al. reported that former and current smokers started smoking e-cigarettes in an attempt to reduce the harm of traditional smoking, and to lessen the exposure of family members and friends to passive smoking [34]. Baweja et al. conducted an online survey on the use of e-cigarettes and the views of experienced users. The authors noted that e-cigarette was mostly used to quit or reduce smoking and to improve overall health. Users reported "taking fewer puffs per session" than conventional smokers [35]. Kim et al. found that never smokers who were exposed to e-cigarette advertisements perceived a lower risk of smoking than those who were exposed to control advertisements [36].

Impact of E-Cigarette Use on Cessation or Reduction of Smoking

Despite the strong belief that e-cigarette use can help reduce or quit smoking, there is a marked variation in self-reported abstinence or reduction rates among smokers who started using e-cigarettes. Bullen et al. investigated the short-term effects of using an e-nicotine delivery device (ENDD) on the desire to smoke in 40 adult smokers. The results showed that those who smoked ENDD containing 16 mg of nicotine for 60 min had 0.82 units less desire to smoke in comparison to the placebo ENDD [37]. In a prospective study on the impact of e-cigarette use on smoking habits, Polosa et al. reported sustained abstinence from smoking in 22.5%, and sustained 50% reduction in smoking in almost one-third (32.5%) of their study group. Their study group, which consisted of 40 subjects, was evaluated 24 weeks after having started e-cigarettes [38]. Using a survey, Siegel et al. examined the effect of e-cigarettes (a particular brand) on quitting smoking and found that two-thirds of their participants had a decrease in the number of cigarettes smoked, while 31% reported smoking abstinence. Moreover, the number of e-cigarettes used per day had an impact on smoking cessation. Those who smoked more than 20 per day had a quit rate of 70% [39]. Caponneto et al. evaluated the effect of e-cigarettes on smoking cessation in 300 smokers who were randomized into three groups according to the concentration of nicotine in the used e-cigarette cartridges. At week 52, complete abstinence documented by eCO test was noted in 8.7% of the cases, and a reduction in smoking was reported in 10.3% of the cases [40]. In a worldwide survey on 19,000 consumers, Farsalinos et al. reported that 81% of former smokers succeeded in substituting cigarettes with e-cigarettes. The authors also noted that e-cigarette use had helped current smokers reduce the number of cigarettes per day. The authors concluded that e-cigarettes are an effective means for cessation of traditional smoking and can be used as a long-term substitute [34]. Biener and Hargraves examined the association between e-cigarette use and smoking cessation or motivation to quit smoking in a cohort of 1374 cigarette smokers, half of whom were followed for 3 years. Regression analysis showed that intense users of e-cigarettes, i.e., those who smoked e-cigarettes daily for at least 1 month, were more likely to report smoking cessation than non-users, with an odds ratio of 6.07 (95% CI) [41]. Lindson et al. conducted a systematic review on the effectiveness of e-cigarettes in helping to quit smoking and noted that nicotine e-cigarette was associated with high quit rates in comparison to other nicotine replacement therapies with high-certainty evidence (RR 1.59, 95% CI). Moreover, there was moderate-certainty evidence that nicotine e-cigarettes also resulted in increased quit rates as compared to non-nicotine e-cigarettes (RR 1.46, 95% CI) [42].

On the other hand, other studies debated the hypothesis that vaping is a significant means to quit smoking. Bullen et al. conducted a randomized controlled study (RCT) that included 657 smokers who had the intent to quit smoking. The study group was divided into three subgroups, each receiving a different treatment regimen, which included behavioral support in addition to either 16-mg nicotine e-cigarettes, 21-mg nicotine patches, or a placebo. Abstinence rate was assessed at 6 months using the eCO test. E-cigarette users had a higher abstinence rate compared to those who used nicotine patches or placebo (7.3% vs.5.8% vs. 4.1%, respectively); however, there was no statistically sufficient power to assert the superiority of e-cigarettes with nicotine to placebo e-cigarettes [43]. Brose et al. investigated the association between e-cigarette use, smoking cessation, smoking cessation attempts, and a decrease in cigarette consumption using a wide-based survey, which included 4064 adult smokers, 43% of whom were followed up for 1 year. The results showed that at baseline, daily use of e-cigarettes succeeded in increasing the rate of attempting to stop smoking and in reducing smoking, but on follow-up, it did not succeed in smoking cessation. On follow-up, the odds of smoking reduction were 2.49 for daily e-cigarette users. Non-daily use of e-cigarettes did not affect smoking habits in terms of decrease or cessation of smoking [44]. Kalkhoran and Glantz conducted a systematic review and meta-analysis on the link between e-cigarettes and smoking cessation and noted that e-cigarette users were less likely to quit cigarettes compared to non-e-cigarette users. The odds ratio of quitting cigarettes in e-cigarette smokers was 0.72, 95% CI. The review, which included 38 studies, 20 of which used controls, concluded that the use of e-cigarettes among smokers was associated with less quitting [45]. Hirano et al. conducted a survey to assess the impact of e-cigarette use and other smoking cessation methods on smoking abstinence. Among the 798 persons who were analyzed, the authors noted a negative association between e-cigarette use and smoking cessation with an odds ratio of

0.632. The authors concluded that e-cigarette use is not very efficacious in smoking cessation among Japanese smokers [46].

References

1. Rom O, Pecorelli A, Valacchi G, Reznick AZ. Are E-cigarettes a safe and good alternative to cigarette smoking? Ann N Y Acad Sci. 2015;1340:65–74. https://doi.org/10.1111/nyas.12609. Epub 2014 Dec 31. PMID: 25557889.
2. Fuoco FC, Buonanno G, Stabile L, Vigo P. Influential parameters on particle concentration and size distribution in the mainstream of e-cigarettes. Environ Pollut. 2014;184:523–9. https://doi.org/10.1016/j.envpol.2013.10.010. Epub 2013 Oct 27. PMID: 24172659.
3. Dinakar C, O'Connor GT. The health effects of electronic cigarettes. N Engl J Med. 2016;375(14):1372–81.
4. Schroeder MJ, Hoffman AC. Electronic cigarettes and nicotine clinical pharmacology. Tob Control. 2014;23 Suppl 2(Suppl 2):ii30–5. https://doi.org/10.1136/tobaccocontrol-2013-051469. PMID: 24732160; PMCID: PMC3995273.
5. Harrell MB, Weaver SR, Loukas A, Creamer M, Marti CN, Jackson CD, Heath JW, Nayak P, Perry CL, Pechacek TF, Eriksen MP. Flavored e-cigarette use: characterizing youth, young adult, and adult users. Prev Med Rep. 2016;5:33–40. https://doi.org/10.1016/j.pmedr.2016.11.001. PMID: 27896041; PMCID: PMC5121224.
6. The WHO tobacco free initiative, Geneva, Switzerland. Cited 14 Jul 2014. http://www.who.int/tobacco/communications/statements/eletronic_cigarettes/en/.
7. Debbaneh P, Dhir S, Anderson M, Rivero A. Electronic cigarettes: a narrative review and cohort study of electronic cigarette users in the otolaryngology clinic. Perm J. 2022;26(4):85–93. https://doi.org/10.7812/TPP/22.009. Epub 2022 Oct 3. PMID: 36184759; PMCID: PMC9761286.
8. Gilbert HA, inventor. Smokeless non-tobacco cigarette. 1965. United States patent 3,209,819. April 17, 1963.
9. Popova L, Ling PM. Alternative tobacco product use and smoking cessation: a national study. Am J Public Health. 2013;103(5):923–30. https://doi.org/10.2105/AJPH.2012.301070. Epub 2013 Mar 14. PMID: 23488521; PMCID: PMC3661190.
10. Regan AK, Promoff G, Dube SR, Arrazola R. Electronic nicotine delivery systems: adult use and awareness of the 'e-cigarette' in the USA. Tob Control. 2013;22(1):19–23. https://doi.org/10.1136/tobaccocontrol-2011-050044. Epub 2011 Oct 27. PMID: 22034071.
11. Ma S, Kaareen A, Park H, He Y, Jiang S, Qiu Z, Xie Z, Li D, Chen J, O'Connor RJ, Fong GT, Shang C. How to identify e-cigarette brands available in the United States during 2020–2022: development and usability study. JMIR Form Res. 2024;8:e47570. https://doi.org/10.2196/47570. PMID: 38416562; PMCID: PMC10938231.
12. IBISWorld. E-cigarette Manufacturing in the US—Market Research Report. https://www.ibisworld.com/united-states/industry/e-cigarette-manufacturing/6196/.
13. Cooper SY, Henderson BJ. The impact of electronic nicotine delivery system (ENDS) flavors on nicotinic acetylcholine receptors and nicotine addiction-related behaviors. Molecules. 2020;25(18):4223. https://doi.org/10.3390/molecules25184223. PMID: 32942576; PMCID: PMC7571084.
14. Adkison SE, O'Connor RJ, Bansal-Travers M, Hyland A, Borland R, Yong HH, Cummings KM, McNeill A, Thrasher JF, Hammond D, Fong GT. Electronic nicotine delivery systems: international tobacco control four-country survey. Am J Prev Med. 2013;44(3):207–15.
15. Mirbolouk M, Charkhchi P, Kianoush S, Uddin SMI, Orimoloye OA, Jaber R, Bhatnagar A, Benjamin EJ, Hall ME, DeFilippis AP, Maziak W, Nasir K, Blaha MJ. Prevalence and distribution of e-cigarette use among U.S. adults: behavioral risk factor surveillance system, 2016.

Ann Intern Med. 2018;169(7):429–38. https://doi.org/10.7326/M17-3440. Epub 2018 Aug 28. PMID: 30167658; PMCID: PMC10534294.

16. Wilson FA, Wang Y. Recent findings on the prevalence of e-cigarette use among adults in the U.S. Am J Prev Med. 2017;52(3):385–390. https://doi.org/10.1016/j.amepre.2016.10.029. Epub 2016 Dec 14. PMID: 27988090.
17. Hedman L, Backman H, Stridsman C, Bosson JA, Lundbäck M, Lindberg A, Rönmark E, Ekerljung L. Association of electronic cigarette use with smoking habits, demographic factors, and respiratory symptoms. JAMA Netw Open. 2018;1(3):e180789. https://doi.org/10.1001/jamanetworkopen.2018.0789. PMID: 30646032; PMCID: PMC6324524.
18. Miech R, Patrick ME, O'Malley PM, Johnston LD. E-cigarette use as a predictor of cigarette smoking: results from a 1-year follow-up of a national sample of 12th grade students. Tob Control. 2017;26(e2):e106–11. https://doi.org/10.1136/tobaccocontrol-2016-053291. Epub 2017 Feb 6. PMID: 28167683; PMCID: PMC5545162.
19. Morean ME, Bold KW, Kong G, Gueorguieva R, Camenga DR, Simon P, Jackson A, Cavallo DA, Krishnan-Sarin S. Adolescents' awareness of the nicotine strength and e-cigarette status of JUUL e-cigarettes. Drug Alcohol Depend. 2019;204:107512.
20. Yoong SL, Stockings E, Chai LK, Tzelepis F, Wiggers J, Oldmeadow C, Paul C, Peruga A, Kingsland M, Attia J, Wolfenden L. Prevalence of electronic nicotine delivery systems (ENDS) use among youth globally: a systematic review and meta-analysis of country level data. Aust N Z J Public Health. 2018;42(3):303–8.
21. Yoong SL, Hall A, Leonard A, McCrabb S, Wiggers J, d'Espaignet ET, Stockings E, Gouda H, Fayokun R, Commar A, Prasad VM. Prevalence of electronic nicotine delivery systems and electronic non-nicotine delivery systems in children and adolescents: a systematic review and meta-analysis. Lancet Public Health. 2021;6(9):e661–73.
22. Boakye E, Osuji N, Erhabor J, Obisesan O, Osei AD, Mirbolouk M, Stokes AC, Dzaye O, El Shahawy O, Hirsch GA, Benjamin EJ. Assessment of patterns in e-cigarette use among adults in the US, 2017–2020. JAMA Netw Open. 2022;5(7):e2223266.
23. Auf R, Trepka MJ, Selim M, Ben Taleb Z, De La Rosa M, Cano MÁ. E-cigarette marketing exposure and combustible tobacco use among adolescents in the United States. Addict Behav. 2018;78:74–9. https://doi.org/10.1016/j.addbeh.2017.10.008. Epub 2017 Oct 14. PMID: 29127787.
24. Mantey DS, Cooper MR, Clendennen SL, Pasch KE, Perry CL. E-cigarette marketing exposure is associated with e-cigarette use among US youth. J Adolesc Health. 2016;58(6):686–90. https://doi.org/10.1016/j.jadohealth.2016.03.003. Epub 2016 Apr 12. PMID: 27080732; PMCID: PMC4900536.
25. Chen-Sankey JC, Unger JB, Bansal-Travers M, Niederdeppe J, Bernat E, Choi K. E-cigarette marketing exposure and subsequent experimentation among youth and young adults. Pediatrics. 2019;144(5):e20191119. https://doi.org/10.1542/peds.2019-1119. PMID: 31659003; PMCID: PMC6836725.
26. Cruz TB, McConnell R, Low BW, Unger JB, Pentz MA, Urman R, Berhane K, Chou CP, Liu F, Barrington-Trimis JL. Tobacco marketing and subsequent use of cigarettes, e-cigarettes, and hookah in adolescents. Nicotine Tob Res. 201921;21(7):926–32. https://doi.org/10.1093/ntr/nty107. PMID: 29846704; PMCID: PMC6588392.
27. Dai L, He Y, Tan Y, Yu Z, Zhu J. Online e-cigarette information exposure and its association with e-cigarette use among adolescents in Shanghai, China. Int J Environ Res Public Health. 2022;19(6):3329. https://doi.org/10.3390/ijerph19063329. PMID: 35329027; PMCID: PMC8949377.
28. Świątkowska B, Zajdel R, Balwicki Ł, Kaleta D. Is e-cigarette advertising associated with e-cigarette use among young people? New survey evidence from Poland. Front Public Health. 2024;12:1448011. https://doi.org/10.3389/fpubh.2024.1448011. PMID: 39435405; PMCID: PMC11491323.
29. Smith MJ, Hilton S. Youth's exposure to and engagement with e-cigarette marketing on social media: a UK focus group study. BMJ Open. 2023;13(8):e071270. https://doi.org/10.1136/bmjopen-2022-071270. PMID: 37612101; PMCID: PMC10450076.

30. Li J, Hui X, Fu J, Ahmed MM, Yao L, Yang K. Electronic cigarettes versus nicotine-replacement therapy for smoking cessation: a systematic review and meta-analysis of randomized controlled trials. Tob Induc Dis. 2022;20:90.
31. Etter JF. Electronic cigarettes: a survey of users. BMC Public Health. 2010;10:1–7.
32. Foulds J, Veldheer S, Berg A. Electronic cigarettes (e-cigs): views of aficionados and clinical/public health perspectives. Int J Clin Pract. 2011;65(10):1037–42. https://doi.org/10.1111/j.1742-1241.2011.02751.x. Epub 2011 Aug 1. PMID: 21801287.
33. Dawkins L, Turner J, Roberts A, Soar K. 'Vaping' profiles and preferences: an online survey of electronic cigarette users. Addiction. 2013;108(6):1115–25. https://doi.org/10.1111/add.12150. Epub 2013 Mar 28. PMID: 23551515.
34. Farsalinos KE, Romagna G, Tsiapras D, Kyrzopoulos S, Voudris V. Characteristics, perceived side effects and benefits of electronic cigarette use: a worldwide survey of more than 19,000 consumers. Int J Environ Res Public Health. 2014;11(4):4356–73. https://doi.org/10.3390/ijerph110404356. PMID: 24758891; PMCID: PMC4025024.
35. Baweja R, Curci KM, Yingst J, Veldheer S, Hrabovsky S, Wilson SJ, Nichols TT, Eissenberg T, Foulds J. Views of experienced electronic cigarette users. Addict Res Theory. 2016;24(1):80–8.
36. Kim M, Popova L, Halpern-Felsher B, Ling PM. Effects of e-cigarette advertisements on adolescents' perceptions of cigarettes. Health Commun. 201;34(3):290–97. https://doi.org/10.1080/10410236.2017.1407230. Epub 2017 Dec 13. PMID: 29236550; PMCID: PMC5999542.
37. Bullen C, McRobbie H, Thornley S, Glover M, Lin R, Laugesen M. Effect of an electronic nicotine delivery device (e cigarette) on desire to smoke and withdrawal, user preferences and nicotine delivery: randomised cross-over trial. Tob Control. 2010;19(2):98–103. https://doi.org/10.1136/tc.2009.031567. PMID: 20378585.
38. Polosa R, Caponnetto P, Morjaria JB, Papale G, Campagna D, Russo C. Effect of an electronic nicotine delivery device (e-Cigarette) on smoking reduction and cessation: a prospective 6-month pilot study. BMC Public Health. 2011;11:786. https://doi.org/10.1186/1471-2458-11-786. PMID: 21989407; PMCID: PMC3203079.
39. Siegel MB, Tanwar KL, Wood KS. Electronic cigarettes as a smoking-cessation: tool results from an online survey. Am J Prev Med. 2011;40(4):472–5. https://doi.org/10.1016/j.amepre.2010.12.006. PMID: 21406283.
40. Caponnetto P, Campagna D, Cibella F, Morjaria JB, Caruso M, Russo C, Polosa R. EffiCiency and Safety of an eLectronic cigAreTte (ECLAT) as tobacco cigarettes substitute: a prospective 12-month randomized control design study. PLoS One. 2013;8(6):e66317. https://doi.org/10.1371/journal.pone.0066317. Erratum in: PLoS One. 2014;9(1).
41. Biener L, Hargraves JL. A longitudinal study of electronic cigarette use among a population-based sample of adult smokers: association with smoking cessation and motivation to quit. Nicotine Tob Res. 2015;17(2):127–33.
42. Lindson N, Butler AR, McRobbie H, Bullen C, Hajek P, Begh R, Theodoulou A, Notley C, Rigotti NA, Turner T, Livingstone-Banks J, Morris T, Hartmann-Boyce J. Electronic cigarettes for smoking cessation. Cochrane Database Syst Rev. 2024;1(1):CD010216. https://doi.org/10.1002/14651858.CD010216.pub8. Update in: Cochrane Database Syst Rev. 2025 Jan 29;1:CD010216. https://doi.org/10.1002/14651858.CD010216.pub9. PMID: 38189560; PMCID: PMC10772980.
43. Bullen C, Howe C, Laugesen M, McRobbie H, Parag V, Williman J, Walker N. Electronic cigarettes for smoking cessation: a randomised controlled trial. Lancet. 2013;382(9905):1629–37.
44. Brose LS, Hitchman SC, Brown J, West R, McNeill A. Is the use of electronic cigarettes while smoking associated with smoking cessation attempts, cessation and reduced cigarette consumption? A survey with a 1-year follow-up. Addiction. 2015;110(7):1160–8. https://doi.org/10.1111/add.12917. Epub 2015 Apr 23. PMID: 25900312; PMCID: PMC4862028.
45. Kalkhoran S, Glantz SA. E-cigarettes and smoking cessation in real-world and clinical settings: a systematic review and meta-analysis. Lancet Respir Med. 2016;4(2):116–28. https://doi.org/10.1016/S2213-2600(15)00521-4. Epub 2016 Jan 14. PMID: 26776875; PMCID: PMC4752870.

46. Hirano T, Tabuchi T, Nakahara R, Kunugita N, Mochizuki-Kobayashi Y. Electronic cigarette use and smoking abstinence in Japan: a cross-sectional study of quitting methods. Int J Environ Res Public Health. 2017;14(2):202. https://doi.org/10.3390/ijerph14020202. PMID: 28218695; PMCID: PMC5334756.

Vaping and Its Adverse Effects on Health 2

Adverse Effects of E-Cigarettes on Health

There is growing concern among healthcare providers about the safety of vaping despite being advertised as a safe smoking habit. More research on the effects of e-cigarettes on health and the hazards of vaping on various systems in the body is coming to the forefront of many discussions. The US General Assembly declared adolescent vaping as an epidemic and highlighted the steps to follow moving forward [1]. The American Academy of Family Physicians highlighted the negative health consequences of vaping and its addictive behavior. The academy also did not advocate the use of electronic nicotine delivery systems (ENDS) as a smoking cessation device [2]. The Centers for Disease Control noted that e-cigarettes are not a safe product and more research is needed to elucidate the long-term effects of vaping [3]. Similarly, based on the Position Statement of the American Academy of Otolaryngology-Head and Neck Surgery, physicians should balance between using e-cigarettes as a means for smoking abstinence and the risk of nicotine addiction when using nicotine-containing e-cigarettes [4]. Last but not least, the American College of Surgeons reported that smoking and vaping before surgery increase the risk of postoperative lung infection and heart attack [5].

All the above position statements are based on cumulative evidence indicating that e-cigarettes affect various systems in the body [6–9]. In 2020, Hua et al. analyzed the health effects associated with e-cigarette smoking using online forum posts. More than 40 thousand posts were analyzed, and the results were consolidated by the system involved and the type of symptoms reported. The systems most commonly affected were the neurologic, respiratory, and digestive systems. For the neurological system, the most common symptoms were headache and fatigue/malaise, followed by nausea and dizziness. For the respiratory system, the most commonly reported symptoms were cough and wheezing, followed by dyspnea. As for the digestive system, the most commonly reported symptoms were heartburn, cramping, and flatus. It is worth noting that some e-cigarette users reported positive

A.-l. Hamdan, *E-Cigarette Smoking, Voice, and Health*,
https://doi.org/10.1007/978-3-032-04913-1_2

symptoms, albeit to a lesser extent than negative symptoms. These included improvement in tiredness, insomnia, wheezing, coughing, and halitosis [6].

There is also growing literature on the impact of e-cigarette use on the cardiovascular system. Carnevale et al. investigated the impact of e-cigarette and traditional cigarette smoking with the same nicotine content on oxidative stress and vascular function in a cohort of 20 smokers who were asked to smoke the two types of cigarettes for 1 week. The blood tests taken after smoking traditional cigarettes and e-cigarettes showed a decrease in vitamin E levels, nitric oxide bioavailability, and flow-mediated dilation, with an increase in soluble NOX2-derived peptide and 8-iso-prostaglandin F2alpha. Although the impact of e-cigarettes on nitric oxide bioavailability and markers of oxidative stress was less than that of traditional cigarettes, there was no significant difference in vitamin E level and flow-mediated dilation between the two groups [9]. Vlachopoulos et al. investigated the acute effect of e-cigarette smoking on blood pressure and aortic stiffness in a cohort of 24 smokers. The participants were examined following the use of traditional cigarettes for 5 min, e-cigarettes for 5 min, e-cigarettes for 30 min, and nothing (sham) for 60 min. Aortic stiffness was measured via the carotid-femoral pulse-wave velocity. The results showed an increase in heart rate by 3.1 beats after 30 min of e-cigarette smoking. Both types of smoking increased the systolic blood pressure. Moreover, e-cigarette smoking for 5 min resulted in an increase in pulse-wave velocity after 15 min and a potent one after the end of smoking. The authors highlighted the implications of their findings on cardiovascular events in e-cigarette smokers [10]. Similarly, Caporale et al. investigated the acute effects of nicotine-free e-cigarette aerosol on vascular function in 31 healthy non-smokers who were evaluated after vaping. The authors reported an increase in resistivity index, an increase in aortic pulse wave velocity, a decrease in hyperemic index, and blunting of luminal flow-mediated dilation [11].

E-cigarette use has also been suggested to play a role in the pathogenesis of malignancies, most common of which are those related to the lungs and bladder. E-cigarette liquid and aerosol contain several toxic substances such as nitrosamines, trace metals, aldehydes, tobacco alkaloids, and polycyclic aromatic hydrocarbons, among other ingredients [12]. Many of these compounds have been associated with reduced cell viability and increased risk of a lifetime cancer [13–15]. Lee et al. examined the DNA damage in mice exposed to e-cigarette smoke and noted tumorigenic transformation and mutational susceptibility of epithelial and urothelial cells. The authors suggested that nicotine nitrosation could be carcinogenic to the murine bladder and lung [16]. Ganapathy et al. examined the genotoxicity of e-cigarette aerosol extracts on oral and lung epithelial cells and noted a dose-dependent DNA damage independent of the nicotine concentration. The damage was less than that observed following exposure to mainstream smoke extracts [17].

Adverse Effects of E-Cigarette Use on Ear, Nose, and Throat

There is ubiquity of reports on the otolaryngologic manifestations of e-cigarette use, with emphasis on the associated symptoms. In a scoping review of 32 studies on the impact of vaping on the ear, nose, and throat, Amanian et al. reported cough as the most common symptom often associated with mouth and throat irritation [18]. Debbaneh et al. reviewed the medical records of 88 e-cigarette users who presented with an ENT complaint. The majority (85.2%) were diagnosed with one inflammatory condition, and 13.5% were diagnosed with two inflammatory conditions. There was no association between inflammatory diagnosis and the duration of smoking [19].

The adverse effects of e-cigarette use on hearing and the vestibular system: The number of studies on the otologic manifestations of vaping is limited. The main reported vestibular symptoms are dizziness and vertigo, with no clear distinction between the two [18]. The vestibular symptoms of e-cigarette use are in line with the known impact of traditional cigarette smoking on the vestibular system. Wada et al. examined the link between traditional cigarette smoking and new peripheral vestibular disorders over 1 year in 393 participants. The results showed that ever smokers, meaning current and past smokers, had a hazard ratio of 2.22 compared to never smokers. The ratio increased to 2.70 when the number of packs per year was equal to or exceeded 30 [20]. Another otologic complaint in e-cigarette users is hearing loss [6]. Many studies suggested an association between smoking and hearing impairment at specific frequencies [21–25]. In a cross-sectional study that included 42,173 participants, Hu et al. noted that exclusive e-cigarette smokers had a higher pooled adjusted odds ratio for unilateral hearing loss at 4 kHz compared to non-smokers (OR 1.46). The odds ratio was lower than that of cigarette smokers and dual smokers (OR 1.83 and 1.66, respectively) [26].

The pathophysiology of hearing impairment secondary to vaping needs further investigation. Based on numerous studies on tobacco smoking and hearing, a suggested mechanism is oxidative damage. Many of the ingredients of e-cigarette liquid and aerosol may be harmful to the auditory system. Nicotine, for instance, has been linked to oxidative stress, inflammation, and dysregulation of the endothelial lining. These can lead to vasoconstriction and impairment of the microcirculation of the inner ear and hair cells [23, 27, 28]. Similarly, carbon monoxide can reduce oxyhemoglobin breakdown and oxygen transfer, further jeopardizing oxygenation of the inner ear structures [29, 30]. Another pathogenic pathway for tobacco-induced hearing impairment is alteration in neural transmission and auditory processing as a result of brainstem involvement. In a review on hearing of smokers, Cavallieri et al. noted an increase in wave I and wave V latency in smokers [31].

The adverse effects of e-cigarette use on the nose and paranasal sinuses: The nose and paranasal sinuses play a major role in regulating air temperature and humidity during inspiration and in filtering inhaled pollutants. Numerous studies in the literature indicate a higher prevalence of symptoms of sinus disease in e-cigarette users in comparison to non-smokers, and that e-cigarette smoking increases the risk of chronic rhinosinusitis (CRS) and allergic rhinitis (AR) [32–35]. Using the

SNOT-22 questionnaire, Kumral et al. reported a high score in e-cigarette users, which decreased after cessation of smoking. Notably, the SNOT-22 score was comparable to that of conventional smokers [32]. In another study, which included 38,413 participants, Rha et al. reported a significant association between e-cigarette use, CRS, and AR. The adjusted odds ratio for CRS and AR in e-cigarette users was 1.38 [34].

The pathophysiology of sinus disease in e-cigarette users is complex and multifaceted. Mechanisms have been suggested, including impairment in muco-ciliary clearance, inflammation, and alteration in the function of the immune system. All these mechanisms can act in concert to increase the risk of bacterial colonization and infection. More information on the impact of e-cigarette use on the nose and paranasal sinuses, and the pathophysiology of sinonasal symptoms in vapors, is available in Chap. 7 of this book.

The adverse effects of e-cigarette use on the larynx and voice: There are only a few reports in the literature on the laryngeal manifestations of vaping, with controversial results. In a study on the adverse effects of e-cigarette use on health using online forum posts, Hua et al. noted a harsh voice as one of the many reported symptoms. Several risk factors for dysphonia were discussed in that study, including dehydration, cough, and infection such as pharyngitis [6]. On the other hand, in a cross-sectional study that included 81 healthy volunteers, Tuhanioglu et al. reported no significant difference in self-reported voice handicap score in e-cigarette users vs. controls. However, the conventional cigarette smoker group had a significantly higher mean VHI-10 score than the e-cigarette group and controls. The higher voice handicap in conventional smokers was substantiated by an elevated shimmer, which refers to cycle-to-cycle variation in intensity [36]. More information on voice disorders in e-cigarette users is available to the readers in Chap. 5 of this book.

Risk of head and neck cancer in e-cigarette users: The risk of head and neck cancer in e-cigarette users is a subject of thorough discussion in the literature. Nguyen et al. reported two cases of oral carcinoma, namely basaloid squamous cell carcinoma, in healthy individuals who consumed 20–30 e-cigarettes per day for 13 years. The authors suggested an association between e-cigarette use and oral cancer [37]. On the other hand, Bardellini et al. reported no significant difference in the total prevalence of pre-cancerous oral mucosal lesions between current e-cigarette users and former tobacco users. Their prospective control study included 90 patients, half of whom were e-cigarette users and the other half were former smokers [38]. Franco et al. reported no significant difference in the number of micronuclei in oral mucosa scrapings of e-cigarette smokers compared to healthy controls. The study was conducted on 65 subjects who were divided into three groups: conventional smokers, e-cigarette smokers, and non-smokers. In conclusion, the authors suggested that the use of e-cigarettes is safe for oral cancer and may have a role in the primary prevention of oral cavity cancer [39].

The mechanisms behind a possible increased risk of head and neck cancer in e-cigarette smokers include cytotoxicity, oxidative stress, decrease in cell viability, and possible DNA damage [40–42]. Flach et al. conducted a systematic review on the possible etiologic role of e-cigarette use in the pathogenesis of head and neck cancer and noted various degrees of oxidative stress and DNA damage [43]. In an in vitro study using pharyngeal mucosal cells that were incubated with flavored e-liquids, Welz et al. noted a decrease in cell viability. Moreover, there was a significant DNA fragmentation following incubation with fruit-flavored liquids [41]. Yu et al. reported cell death and DNA double-strand breaks in epithelial cell lines following exposure to e-cigarettes. The authors also noted a significant reduction in cell viability and an increased rate of apoptosis irrespective of the vapor nicotine content [44]. Korrapati et al. reported an increase in the death of normal epithelial cells following treatment with e-cigarette aerosol, ranging from 24 h to 4 weeks. The increase in cell death was higher when an e-cigarette with nicotine was used (10 times vs. 5 times, respectively) [45]. Bustamante et al. reported the presence of an endogenous oral and esophageal carcinogen N′-nitrosonornicotine (NNN) in the saliva of e-cigarette users. Despite the well-known carcinogenic potency of NNN, the potential risk of this carcinogen in e-cigarette smokers remains unclear and needs further investigation [46].

References

1. Farzal Z, Perry MF, Yarbrough WG, Kimple AJ. The adolescent vaping epidemic in the United States-how it happened and where we go from here. JAMA Otolaryngol Head Neck Surg. 2019;145(10):885–6. https://doi.org/10.1001/jamaoto.2019.2410. PMID: 31436792
2. American Academy of Family Physicians. Electronic nicotine delivery systems (ENDS) [Internet]. Leawood (KS): AAFP; [cited 2025 Apr 30]. https://www.aafp.org/about/policies/all/electronic-nicotine-delivery-systems.html.
3. Centers for Disease Control and Prevention. Electronic cigarettes [Internet]. Atlanta (GA): CDC; [updated 2024 Apr 2; cited 2025 Apr 29]. https://www.cdc.gov/tobacco/e-cigarettes/index.html.
4. American Academy of Otolaryngology–Head and Neck Surgery. Position statements on e-cigarettes [Internet]. Alexandria (VA): AAO-HNS; [cited 2025 Apr 30]. https://www.entnet.org/resource/position-statements-on-e-cigarettes/.
5. American College of Surgeons. American College of Surgeons panels warn vaping and marijuana use before an operation can be harmful [Internet]. Chicago (IL): ACS; 2020 [cited 2025 Apr 30]. https://www.facs.org/media-center/press-releases/2020/smoking100620/.
6. Hua M, Sadah S, Hristidis V, Talbot P. Health effects associated with electronic cigarette use: automated mining of online forums. J Med Internet Res. 2020;22(1):e15684.
7. King JL, Reboussin BA, Wiseman KD, Ribisl KM, Seidenberg AB, Wagoner KG, Wolfson M, Sutfin EL. Adverse symptoms users attribute to e-cigarettes: results from a national survey of US adults. Drug Alcohol Depend. 2019;196:9–13. https://doi.org/10.1016/j.drugalcdep.2018.11.030. Epub 2019 Jan 11. PMID: 30658221; PMCID: PMC6377331.
8. King JL, Reboussin BA, Merten JW, Wiseman KD, Wagoner KG, Sutfin EL. Negative health symptoms reported by youth e-cigarette users: results from a national survey of US youth. Addict Behav. 2020;104:106315. https://doi.org/10.1016/j.addbeh.2020.106315. Epub 2020 Jan 13. PMID: 31981796; PMCID: PMC8055041.
9. Carnevale R, Sciarretta S, Violi F, Nocella C, Loffredo L, Perri L, Peruzzi M, Marullo AG, De Falco E, Chimenti I, Valenti V. Acute impact of tobacco vs electronic cigarette smoking on oxidative stress and vascular function. Chest. 2016;150(3):606–12.
10. Vlachopoulos C, Ioakeimidis N, Abdelrasoul M, Terentes-Printzios D, Georgakopoulos C, Pietri P, Stefanadis C, Tousoulis D. Electronic cigarette smoking increases aortic stiffness and blood pressure in young smokers. J Am Coll Cardiol. 2016;67(23):2802–3.

11. Caporale A, Langham MC, Guo W, Johncola A, Chatterjee S, Wehrli FW. Acute effects of electronic cigarette aerosol inhalation on vascular function detected at quantitative MRI. Radiology. 2019;293(1):97–106. https://doi.org/10.1148/radiol.2019190562. Epub 2019 Aug 20. PMID: 31429679; PMCID: PMC6776371.
12. Goniewicz ML, Knysak J, Gawron M, Kosmider L, Sobczak A, Kurek J, Prokopowicz A, Jablonska-Czapla M, Rosik-Dulewska C, Havel C, Jacob P 3rd, Benowitz N. Levels of selected carcinogens and toxicants in vapour from electronic cigarettes. Tob Control. 2014;23(2):133–9. https://doi.org/10.1136/tobaccocontrol-2012-050859. Epub 2013 Mar 6. PMID: 23467656; PMCID: PMC4154473.
13. Gaur S, Agnihotri R. Health effects of trace metals in electronic cigarette aerosols—a systematic review. Biol Trace Elem Res. 2019;188(2):295–315. https://doi.org/10.1007/s12011-018-1423-x. Epub 2018 Jul 4. PMID: 29974385.
14. Jensen RP, Luo W, Pankow JF, Strongin RM, Peyton DH. Hidden formaldehyde in e-cigarette aerosols. N Engl J Med. 2015;372(4):392–4. https://doi.org/10.1056/NEJMc1413069. PMID: 25607446.
15. Zborovskaya Y. E-cigarettes and smoking cessation: a primer for oncology clinicians. Clin J Oncol Nurs. 2017;21(1):54–63. https://doi.org/10.1188/17.CJON.54-63. PMID: 28107337.
16. Lee HW, Park SH, Weng MW, Wang HT, Huang WC, Lepor H, Wu XR, Chen LC, Tang MS. E-cigarette smoke damages DNA and reduces repair activity in mouse lung, heart, and bladder as well as in human lung and bladder cells. Proc Natl Acad Sci. 2018;115(7):E1560–9.
17. Ganapathy V, Manyanga J, Brame L, McGuire D, Sadhasivam B, Floyd E, Rubenstein DA, Ramachandran I, Wagener T, Queimado L. Electronic cigarette aerosols suppress cellular antioxidant defenses and induce significant oxidative DNA damage. PLoS One. 2017;12(5):e0177780. https://doi.org/10.1371/journal.pone.0177780. PMID: 28542301; PMCID: PMC5436899.
18. Amanian A, Phulka J, Hu AC. Unintended side effects of electronic cigarettes in otolaryngology: a scoping review. Otolaryngol Head Neck Surg. 2023;168(1):7–13.
19. Debbaneh P, Dhir S, Anderson M, Rivero A. Electronic cigarettes: a narrative review and cohort study of electronic cigarette users in the otolaryngology clinic. Perm J. 2022;26(4):85.
20. Wada M, Takeshima T, Nakamura Y, Nagasaka S, Kamesaki T, Kajii E, Kotani K. Association between smoking and the peripheral vestibular disorder: a retrospective cohort study. Sci Rep. 2017;7(1):16889.
21. Palmer KT, Griffin MJ, Syddall HE, Coggon D. Cigarette smoking, occupational exposure to noise, and self reported hearing difficulties. Occup Environ Med. 2004;61(4):340–4.
22. Jedrzejczak WW, Koziel M, Kochanek K, Skarzynski H. Otoacoustic emissions in smoking and nonsmoking young adults. Clin Exp Otorhinolaryngol. 2015;8(4):303.
23. Kumar A, Gulati R, Singhal S, Hasan A, Khan A. The effect of smoking on the hearing status—a hospital based study. J Clin Diagn Res. 2013;7(2):210.
24. Rogha M, Hashemi M, Askari N, Abtahi SH, Sepehrnejad M, Nilforoush MH. Cigarette smoking effect on human cochlea responses. Adv Biomed Res. 2015;4(1):148.
25. Sumit AF, Das A, Sharmin Z, Ahsan N, Ohgami N, Kato M, Akhand AA. Cigarette smoking causes hearing impairment among Bangladeshi population. PLoS One. 2015;10(3):e0118960.
26. Hu H, Miyake H, Kochi T, Miyamoto T, Okazaki H, Kabe I, Tomizawa A, Nakagawa T, Honda T, Yamamoto S, Konishi M. Association of conventional cigarette smoking, heated tobacco product use, and dual use with hearing loss: a working population-based study. Tob Induc Dis. 2024;22:10–8332.
27. Schweitzer KS, Chen SX, Law S, Van Demark M, Poirier C, Justice MJ, Hubbard WC, Kim ES, Lai X, Wang M, Kranz WD. Endothelial disruptive proinflammatory effects of nicotine and e-cigarette vapor exposures. Am J Physiol Lung Cell Mol Physiol. 2015;309:L175.
28. El-Mahdy MA, Abdelghany TM, Hemann C, Ewees MG, Mahgoup EM, Eid MS, Shalaan MT, Alzarie YA, Zweier JL. Chronic cigarette smoke exposure triggers a vicious cycle of leukocyte and endothelial-mediated oxidant stress that results in vascular dysfunction. Am J Phys Heart Circ Phys. 2020;319(7):H51–65.

29. Téllez J, Rodríguez A. Carbon monoxide contamination: an environmental health problem. Rev Salud Pública. 2006;8(1):108–17.
30. Ferreira DG, Oliveira GL, Meira AL, Lacerda A. Auditory effects of combined exposure: interaction between carbon monoxide, noise and smoking. Rev Soc Bras Fonoaudiol. 2012;17:405–11.
31. Cavallieri GV, Alcarás PA, Corazza MC, Corazza LA. The hearing of smokers: a review. Revista CEFAC. 2017;19:406–16.
32. Kumral TL, Saltürk Z, Yildirim G, Uyar Y, Berkiten G, Atar Y, Inan M. How does electronic cigarette smoking affect sinonasal symptoms and nasal mucociliary clearance? B-ENT. 2016;12(1):17–21.
33. Pingree G, DeShazo J, Schuman T. Impact of dual electronic and conventional cigarette use on diagnosis and surgery for chronic rhinosinusitis: a multicenter study. Int Forum Allergy Rhinol. 2024;14(5):977–80.
34. Rha MS, Cho HJ, Yoon JH, Kim CH. Association between the use of electronic cigarettes and the prevalence of chronic rhinosinusitis and allergic rhinitis: a nationwide cross-sectional study. Rhinology. 2022;60(1):20–8.
35. Chung SJ, Kim BK, Oh JH, Shim JS, Chang YS, Cho SH, Yang MS. Novel tobacco products including electronic cigarette and heated tobacco products increase risk of allergic rhinitis and asthma in adolescents: analysis of Korean youth survey. Allergy. 2020;75(7):1640–8.
36. Tuhanioğlu B, Erkan SO, Özdaş T, Derici Ç, Tüzün K, Şenkal ÖA. The effect of electronic cigarettes on voice quality. J Voice. 2019;33(5):811.e13–7. https://doi.org/10.1016/j.jvoice.2018.03.015. Epub 2018 Jun 5. PMID: 29884511.
37. Nguyen H, Kitzmiller JP, Nguyen KT, Nguyen C, Bui T. Oral carcinoma associated with chronic use of electronic cigarettes. Otolaryngol (Sunnyvale). 2017;7(2):304.
38. Bardellini E, Amadori F, Conti G, Majorana A. Oral mucosal lesions in electronic cigarettes consumers versus former smokers. Acta Odontol Scand. 2018;76(3):226–8. https://doi.org/10.1080/00016357.2017.1406613. Epub 2017 Nov 21. PMID: 29161938.
39. Franco T, Trapasso S, Puzzo L, Allegra E. Electronic cigarette: role in the primary prevention of oral cavity cancer. Clin Med Insights Ear Nose Throat. 2016:CMENT-S40364
40. Song JJ, Go YY, Mun JY, Lee S, Im GJ, Kim YY, Lee JH, Chang J. Effect of electronic cigarettes on human middle ear. Int J Pediatr Otorhinolaryngol. 2018;109:67–71. https://doi.org/10.1016/j.ijporl.2018.03.028. Epub 2018 Mar 28. PMID: 29728187.
41. Welz C, Canis M, Schwenk-Zieger S, Becker S, Stucke V, Ihler F, Baumeister P. Cytotoxic and genotoxic effects of electronic cigarette liquids on human mucosal tissue cultures of the oropharynx. J Environ Pathol Toxicol Oncol. 2016;35(4):343–54. https://doi.org/10.1615/JEnvironPatholToxicolOncol.2016016652. PMID: 27992314.
42. Sundar IK, Javed F, Romanos GE, Rahman I. E-cigarettes and flavorings induce inflammatory and pro-senescence responses in oral epithelial cells and periodontal fibroblasts. Oncotarget. 2016;7(47):77196–204.
43. Flach S, Maniam P, Manickavasagam J. E-cigarettes and head and neck cancers: a systematic review of the current literature. Clin Otolaryngol. 2019;44(5):749–56.
44. Yu V, Rahimy M, Korrapati A, Xuan Y, Zou AE, Krishnan AR, Tsui T, Aguilera JA, Advani S, Crotty Alexander LE, Brumund KT, Wang-Rodriguez J, Ongkeko WM. Electronic cigarettes induce DNA strand breaks and cell death independently of nicotine in cell lines. Oral Oncol. 2016;52:58–65. https://doi.org/10.1016/j.oraloncology.2015.10.018. Epub 2015 Nov 4. PMID: 26547127; PMCID: PMC4891196.
45. Korrapati A, Yu V, Saad MA, Rahimy M, Xuan Y, Zou A, Krishnan A, Brumund K, Ongkeko WM. The carcinogenic effects of electronic cigarettes in oral cancer. Cancer Res. 2016;76(14_Suppl):4069.
46. Bustamante G, Ma B, Yakovlev G, Yershova K, Le C, Jensen J, Hatsukami DK, Stepanov I. Presence of the carcinogen N′-nitrosonornicotine in saliva of e-cigarette users. Chem Res Toxicol. 2018;31(8):731–8.

Part II

The Phonatory System

3 Anatomy and Physiology of Phonation

Clinical Anatomy of the Larynx

Laryngeal Skeleton

The larynx is a semi-tubular structure with three main rigid components: the hyoid bone, the thyroid cartilage, and the cricoid cartilage (Fig. 3.1). The hyoid bone is a U-shaped structure linked to the styloid process posteriorly via the stylohyoid ligament. Its attachment to the base of the skull provides stability to the suspended laryngeal framework. The hyoid bone also acts as an anchor for the strap muscles, providing agility in swallowing, phonation, and breathing. Below the hyoid bone is the thyroid cartilage. The thyroid cartilage is the largest cartilage in the larynx. It consists of two thyroid lamina that diverge anteriorly at an angle of 90° in men and 120° in women. This cross-gender difference is important to note in laryngeal framework surgery. Each thyroid lamina extends posteriorly and forms the superior and inferior cornu [1]. The superior cornu connects with the hyoid bone via the thyrohyoid ligament, and the inferior cornu connects with the cricoid cartilage via the cricothyroid joint posteriorly, and the cricothyroid ligament anteriorly. The most prominent part of the thyroid cartilage in the neck is labeled "Adam's Apple" (Fig. 3.2). Superior to it is a V-shaped groove, the thyroid notch (Fig. 3.1). The thyroid notch is an important anatomic landmark to identify while performing injection laryngoplasty using the thyrohyoid approach [2]. Another consideration to note is the ossification of the thyroid cartilage, which can start early in life and progress with age [3]. An ossified thyroid cartilage may prohibit the use of the transthyroid approach in injection laryngoplasty. Underneath the thyroid cartilage is a circumferential structure, the cricoid cartilage. The luminal cross-section of the cricoid cartilage is the narrowest of the upper airway and varies with gender and age. It ranges between 8.9 and 17.0 mm in women and between 11.0 and 21.5 mm in men [4]. The cricoid cartilage harbors the posterior cricoarytenoid muscles on its posterior facet,

A.-l. Hamdan, *E-Cigarette Smoking, Voice, and Health*,
https://doi.org/10.1007/978-3-032-04913-1_3

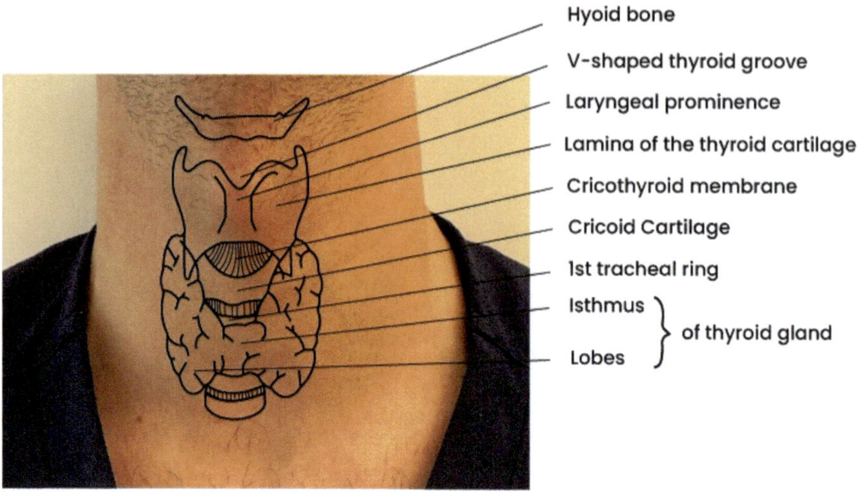

Fig. 3.1 Scheme describing the anatomical landmarks of the larynx

the height of which is around 30 mm. Anteriorly, the cricoid cartilage forms a thin arch to which the cricothyroid muscles and membranes attach (Fig. 3.1).

Other important cartilaginous structures in the larynx include the arytenoid cartilages and the epiglottis (Fig. 3.3). The arytenoid cartilages are pyramidal structures that sit on top of the cricoid cartilage. Each has a muscular process, a vocal process, and an apex. These processes provide attachments to the adductor and abductor muscles. Contraction of these muscles allows the arytenoid cartilages to rotate, glide, and rock. The backward rotatory movement of the arytenoid cartilages allows widening of the glottic aperture, whereas the forward and anterior movement allows closure of the glottic aperture. The epiglottis is a leaf-shaped fibroelastic cartilage attached superiorly to the hyoid bone via the hyo-epiglottic ligament and inferiorly to the thyroid cartilage via the thyro-epiglottic ligament. The most inferior and thinnest part is called the petiole (Fig. 3.3). The petiole is the desired site of entry to the laryngeal inlet using the thyrohyoid approach in injection laryngoplasty. The epiglottis plays a crucial role in protecting the airway during swallowing. The anterior and cephalic movement of the hyoid bone during the initial phase of swallowing pulls the hyo-epiglottic ligament, resulting in folding of the epiglottic cartilage toward the laryngeal inlet. This folding protects the airway and helps prevent aspiration.

Other less important cartilages in the larynx include the corniculate cartilages and the cuneiform cartilages. The corniculate cartilages are located on top of the arytenoid cartilages, whereas the cuneiform cartilages are situated in the aryepiglottic folds. These cartilages provide more rigidity to the aryepiglottic fold during the folding and unfolding that occurs during deglutition [5–7].

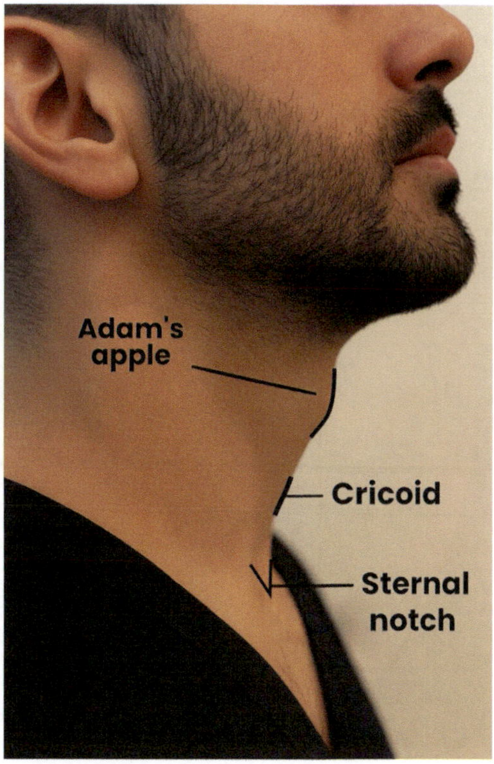

Fig. 3.2 Scheme describing the sagittal view of the anatomical landmarks of the larynx

Laryngeal Extrinsic Muscles

The larynx is a suspended structure in the neck, held in place by various muscles, most important of which are the extrinsic laryngeal muscles. These muscles play a major role in balancing the cephalo-caudal position of the larynx and can be stratified as suprahyoid and infrahyoid muscles. The suprahyoid muscles consist of the stylohyoid, digastric, mylohyoid, and geniohyoid muscles. These muscles act as elevators of the laryngeal skeleton. The mylohyoid muscle, for instance, elevates and pulls the hyoid bone anteriorly, whereas the stylohyoid muscle elevates and pulls the hyoid bone posteriorly [8, 9]. Hyperactivity of the suprahyoid muscles results in a high-positioned larynx. A high-positioned larynx and stiffness in the submental area are signs of muscle tension dysphonia. Another cause for an elevated larynx is a decrease in respiratory capacity. Patients with a low lung volume may exhibit cephalic displacement of the larynx [10]. The infrahyoid muscles consist of the thyrohyoid, sternohyoid, and sternothyroid muscles. These muscles act as laryngeal depressors. The contraction of the sternothyroid and sternohyoid muscles results in lowering the thyroid cartilage and hyoid bone, respectively, whereas contraction of the thyrohyoid muscle results in shortening of the distance between the

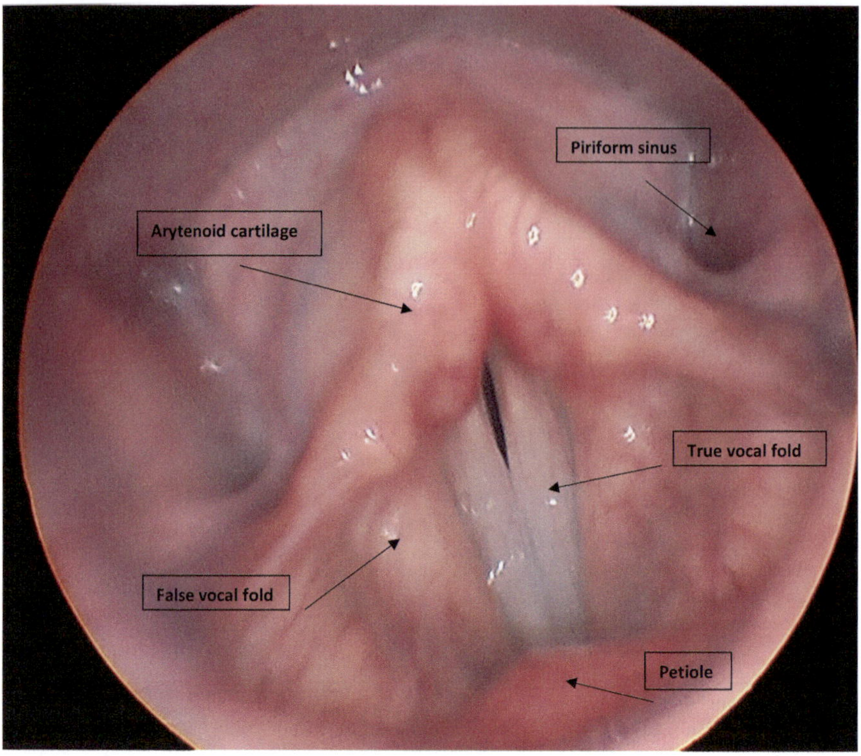

Fig. 3.3 Endoscopic view of the larynx showing laryngeal anatomy when vocal folds are in adduction

thyroid cartilage and hyoid bone. Narrowing of the space between these two structures is also a sign of laryngeal tension in patients with muscle tension dysphonia.

The extrinsic laryngeal muscles also play a major role in modulating the vocal tract dimensions. An elevation of the larynx results in shortening of the vocal tract. Shortening the distance between the lips and vocal folds increases the formants' position, whereas lengthening of the vocal tract results in lowering of the formants and an increase in their dispersion [11].

Intrinsic Laryngeal Muscles

The intrinsic laryngeal muscles play a major role in phonation. These include the thyroarytenoid muscles, the lateral cricoarytenoid muscles, the inter-arytenoid muscles, the cricothyroid muscles, and the posterior cricoarytenoid muscles. A disturbance in any of the intrinsic laryngeal muscles can lead to a voice or breathing disorder.

The thyroarytenoid muscles: The thyroarytenoid (TA) muscle makes up most of the bulk of the vocal fold. It originates anteriorly from the posterior and inferior surface of the thyroid lamina and inserts into the vocal process of the arytenoid cartilage. The TA muscle adducts, lowers, and shortens the vocal fold by drawing the arytenoid cartilage closer to the thyroid cartilage. By doing so, the tension within the vocal fold decreases, and the mass per unit length increases. For that reason, the TA muscle is labeled as a pitch-lowering muscle. During its contraction, the body stiffens, whereas the cover becomes slack, allowing more vibration of the vocal fold cover [12, 13].

The lateral cricoarytenoid muscles: The lateral cricoarytenoid (LCA) muscle originates from the lateral and anterior cricoid cartilage and inserts into the muscular process of the arytenoid cartilage. When it contracts, it adducts and lowers the vocal fold. By bringing the vocal processes into the midline, it also elongates and thins the vocal folds. Hyperactivity of the LCA muscle has been associated with pathologic conditions such as vocal process granuloma. Increased contraction of the LCA muscle results in an angulation of the junction between the vocal process and the membranous portion of the vocal fold [12].

The inter-arytenoid muscle: The inter-arytenoid (IA) muscle consists of transverse and oblique fibers. The oblique fibers extend from the cricoid cartilage to the apex of the arytenoid, whereas the transverse fibers extend from the lateral margin of one arytenoid to the opposite lateral margin of the contralateral one. The IA muscle plays a role in compressing the posterior glottis by adducting the vocal processes of the vocal folds [12].

The cricothyroid muscles: The cricothyroid muscle originates from the anterior and lateral surface of the cricoid arch and inserts into the thyroid lamina. The vertical belly inserts on the anterior part of the thyroid cartilage, whereas the oblique belly inserts on the posterior part of the thyroid cartilage and also on part of its inferior cornu. The CT muscle acts by shortening the distance between the thyroid and cricoid cartilages. As a result, there is an increase in the distance between the vocal process and the anterior attachment of the TA muscle to the thyroid cartilage. Contraction of the CT muscle leads to elongation and thinning of the vocal fold and hence to an increase in tension. All the layers of the vocal fold are stiffened. Contraction of the CT muscles also contributes to the abduction of the vocal folds by bringing them to the midline [14].

The posterior cricoarytenoid muscles: The posterior cricoarytenoid (PCA) muscle originates from the posterior surface of the cricoid lamina and inserts on the muscular process of the arytenoid cartilage, specifically on its posteroinferior surface. The PCA muscle abducts and elevates the vocal folds. The posterolateral rocking movement of the arytenoid cartilage also results in elongation and thinning of the vocal fold, with stiffening of all its layers [5, 7].

Laryngeal Joints

The two most important joints in the larynx are the cricoarytenoid joint (CAJ) and the cricothyroid joint (CTJ). The cricoarytenoid joints are diarthrodial synovial joints that link the cricoid cartilage to the arytenoid cartilages and support the movement of the arytenoid cartilages on top of the cricoid facet. They allow adduction and abduction of the vocal folds following contraction of the adductors and abductor muscles, respectively. The cricoarytenoid ligaments help stabilize the arytenoid cartilages in place during the movement of the vocal folds. Dysfunction of the CAJ, secondary to trauma or inflammation, as seen in patients with autoimmune diseases, can restrict the mobility of the vocal folds. One example is rheumatoid arthritis, which may lead to ankylosis of the CAJ and fixation of the vocal folds. Early treatment with systemic or intra-articular steroid injection is advocated to halt disease progression [15].

The CTJ is also a diarthrodial joint. It allows both rotation and anterior translocation of the thyroid cartilage upon contraction of the CT muscle [16]. Downward rotation of the thyroid cartilage results in narrowing of the visor angle, with elongation and stretching of the vocal folds. The vocal folds are also thinned and elongated by the anterior displacement of the thyroid cartilage [16].

Neurovascular Supply of the Larynx

The larynx is innervated by the superior and inferior laryngeal nerves, branches of the vagal nerve. The external branch of the superior laryngeal nerve innervates the CT muscle. Although it provides motor innervation of the CT muscle, it is also responsible for sensory innervation of the anterior subglottic region [17, 18]. The internal branch of the superior laryngeal nerve, which enters the larynx at the level of the thyrohyoid membrane posteriorly, is responsible for the chemical, heat, and touch receptors of the supraglottic region. The superior or recurrent laryngeal nerve enters the larynx posteriorly and laterally, and innervates all the rest of the intrinsic laryngeal muscles. The recurrent laryngeal nerve also conveys sensory information from sensory receptors in the subglottic region, thus contributing to the sensory input of the larynx. It is important to note the rich neural anastomosis between the superior and inferior laryngeal nerves [19–21].

The vascular supply of the larynx is provided by the superior laryngeal artery, the inferior laryngeal artery, and the cricothyroid artery. The superior laryngeal artery originates from the superior thyroid artery and enters the larynx through the thyrohyoid membrane posteriorly. It supplies most of the supraglottic structures, such as the epiglottis, the vocal fold mucosa, and the adductor muscles. The inferior laryngeal artery originates from the inferior thyroid artery and supplies the PCA muscle in addition to part of the false vocal folds and ventricles [19]. The cricothyroid artery originates from the superior thyroid artery and supplies some of the extrinsic laryngeal muscles in addition to the CT muscles and part of the subglottic region. The vascular supply to the vocal fold submucosal vessels runs parallel to the long axis of the vocal fold and its vibratory margin, which may contribute to the malleability of the vocal fold cover during phonation. The submucosal vocal fold vessels rarely communicate with the vasculature of the underlying vocalis muscles. Aberrant patterns may be observed more frequently in patients with different vocal fold pathology [22].

Inside View of the Larynx

Mucosal surface: Throughout the respiratory tract, the mucosal lining is pseudostratified ciliated columnar except at the level of the true vocal fold, where the lining is non-keratinizing stratified squamous cell epithelium [23]. This helps the vocal folds withstand the stress of phonation. Another factor that helps mitigate the stress of phonation is hydration. Hydration plays a major role in reducing the phonatory threshold pressure, i.e., the pressure needed to set the vocal folds in vibration. Numerous studies indicate that dehydration, local or systemic, results in an increase in phonatory effort, and that laryngeal desiccation may predispose to functional and structural voice disorders [24–27].

The true vocal folds: The vocal folds are the main oscillators of the larynx. They extend from the arytenoid cartilages posteriorly to the inner surface of the thyroid lamina anteriorly and inferior to the petiole. Based on Hirano's histologic description, the vocal fold consists of a mucosa, lamina propria, and muscles [28]. The mucosa and the superficial layer of the lamina propria represent the cover, the intermediate and deep layers represent the transition, and the vocalis and thyroarytenoid muscles represent the body. This architecture allows the vocal folds' cover to vibrate over the body and provides the anatomic basis for the vertical phase difference during a vibratory cycle (Figs. 3.4 and 3.5).

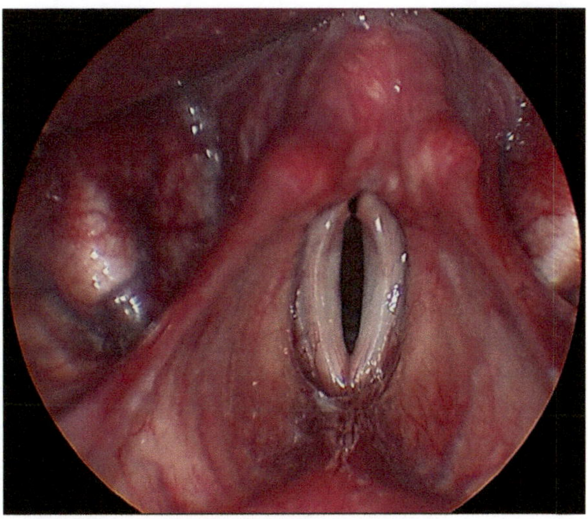

Fig. 3.4 Endoscopic view of the larynx showing the opened phase of a glottic cycle

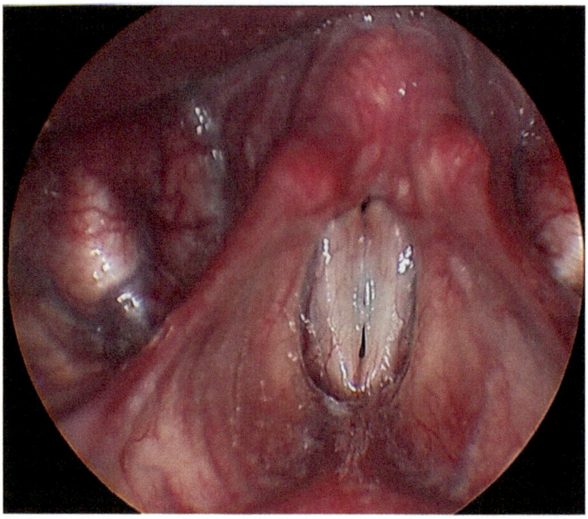

Fig. 3.5 Endoscopic view of the larynx showing the closed phase of a glottic cycle

The false vocal folds: The false vocal folds are the structures situated above the true vocal folds. They are separated from the true vocal folds by the ventricles.

Physiology of Phonation

Phonation is a complex process linked to various systems in the body. It requires a fine interplay between the respiratory and laryngeal muscles, as well as intricate sensory and motor control. The three main components of the phonatory apparatus are the power source, the oscillator, and the resonator.

The power source of phonation: The main power source of voice is the expiratory flow from the lungs. The expiratory flow is supported by the action of the expiratory muscles, namely the abdominal and internal intercostal muscles. Contraction of the expiratory muscles not only helps direct airflow upward but also regulates the subglottic pressure. Chest wall kinematics have shown that changes in rib cage dimensions are associated with alterations in airflow pressure [29]. The back muscles and diaphragm also assist in regulating expiratory flow. The diaphragm, which is a major inspiratory muscle that contributes to more than two-thirds of the lung volume variation during quiet breathing [30], plays a significant role in controlling subglottic pressure during phonation. This is of paramount importance in singers who need to sustain a note and during the transition between vocal registers, particularly when sliding from a high to a low note. Studies have shown that the control of subglottic pressure is accomplished by the differential contraction of various subunits of the diaphragm, which act in concert to adjust the voice signal during performance [29, 31].

The oscillator and the voice source signal: The main oscillator is the vocal folds, although supraglottic structures do play a role in sound production in professional voice users and extreme pathological conditions [32]. It is important to note that sound is produced by the small bursts of air that escape as the vocal folds open and close, and not by the vibration of the vocal folds like that of a string in a musical instrument [33]. The rate of vibration, opening and closing of the vocal folds, also called fundamental frequency, is determined by the glottic airflow and vibratory characteristics of the vocal folds. Based on the body-cover concept described by Hirano et al., there is a vertical phase difference between the upper and lower lip displacement in a glottic cycle. The cover, which consists of the mucosa and superficial layer of the lamina propria, slides over the body during vocal fold vibration [28].

That said, the vibratory glottal cycle consists of several stages. Initially, the vocal folds approximate in the midline and assume a near-total adductor position. This allows the subglottic pressure to increase, resulting in a transglottic pressure gradient. Once the subglottic pressure reaches a certain level, the lower lips of the vocal folds are pushed apart, creating a dome-like configuration. This is followed by further spread of the upper lip, creating a slit aperture. This lateral displacement of the vocal folds, which starts from bottom up, allows the flow of air between the vocal folds. Under the Bernoulli law, this cycle will repeat itself. The narrow opening between the vocal folds increases the speed of the airflow while reducing the pressure on the glottal walls, i.e., the vocal folds' surface. The negative force generated by the Bernoulli effect and the decrease in subglottal pressure as the airstream flows through the glottis result in medial displacement or a pull of the vocal folds to midline. This movement starts with the lower lip and progresses to the upper lip, creating a divergent dome that ends with complete closure of the vocal folds. In turn, this allows the subglottal pressure to build up again, and the cycle repeats itself. The myoelastic properties of the vocal folds also play a role in regulating the closure of the vocal folds and their vibratory behavior. They are partially responsible for the recoil of the vocal folds to the midline after being deflected laterally by the airstream traveling from the trachea upward.

Sound frequency: Sound frequency, the acoustic correlate of voice pitch, is primarily determined by the vocal fold characteristics, namely mass, tension, and length. With an increase in mass per unit length, there is a decrease in voice pitch. In other words, as the vocal folds become heavier, there is a drop in their rate of vibration. An example is Reinke's edema. Patients with Reinke's edema present with deepening of the voice as a result of the increase in mass per unit length [34]. The second determinant of voice pitch is tension. There is a positive correlation between vocal fold tension and pitch. With an increase in vocal fold tension, there is a rise in voice pitch. An example is a patient with vocal fold scarring who often presents with an increase in voice pitch in addition to other voice symptoms [35]. Last is vocal fold length. There is an inverse correlation between the vocal fold length and pitch. One example is the differential growth of the vocal folds at puberty across genders. The longer and heavier vocal folds in men compared to women partially explain the dichotomy in voice pitch. Another example is glottoplasty, a voice feminization procedure that shortens the vocal folds by creating an anterior glottic web [36].

In normal conditions, the voice pitch is regulated by the action of two muscles, referred to as the pitch-regulating muscles, namely the CT and the TA muscles. The cricothyroid muscle has two bellies, a diagonal one and a vertical one. Contraction of the diagonal belly of the CT muscle results in an anterior displacement of the thyroid cartilage. On the other hand, contraction of the vertical belly of the cricothyroid muscle results in downward rotation of the thyroid cartilage along the cricothyroid joint pivot. Both the rocking and rotation movements at the CT joint increase the distance between the arytenoids and thyroid cartilage, resulting in lengthening of the vocal folds. The contraction of the CT muscle also results in thinning of the vocal folds and a decrease in mass per unit length. These morphologic changes lead to an increase in voice pitch (Fig. 3.6). On the other hand, voice pitch decreases by passive relaxation or active contraction of the TA muscle. As the TA muscle contracts, there is approximation of the thyroid and arytenoid cartilages (Fig. 3.7). This shortening in the length of the vocal folds results not only in a decrease in the vocal fold cover tension but also in an increase in mass per unit length of the vocal fold body. Given the inverse relation between vocal fold mass and pitch, there is a further drop in voice pitch.

It is important to note that voice pitch is also affected by airflow and subglottic pressure. An increase in subglottic pressure results in an increase in both pitch and loudness. Professional voice users learn how to dissociate between these two voice characteristics. Using various techniques, including acoustic software, singers train to raise their voice pitch while maintaining the same loudness. This is of paramount importance in performing a passagio from the low note to the high one [37].

Sound amplitude: Sound during phonation is produced by the bursts of air emitted as the vocal folds open and close abruptly. The most important determinant of sound intensity, the acoustic correlate of loudness, is the subglottic pressure. The minimum subglottic pressure needed to set the vocal folds in vibration, or to start a glottal cycle, is the phonatory threshold pressure (PTP). For the speaking voice, PTP is estimated to be on average 7 cm of water [5]. With an increase in subglottal pressure, there is an increase in loudness [33]. Another determinant of sound intensity is the extent of glottic closure. Patients with hyperadduction of the vocal folds

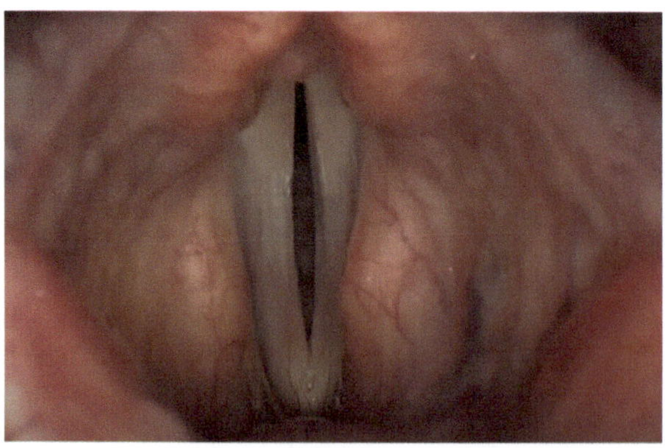

Fig. 3.6 Endoscopic view of the larynx showing the vocal folds during high-pitch phonation

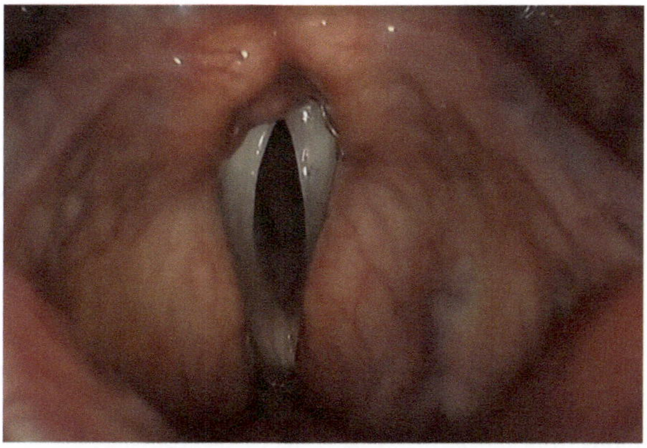

Fig. 3.7 Endoscopic view of the larynx showing the vocal folds during low-pitch phonation

and a high subglottic pressure have difficulty projecting their voice. The term pressed phonation is commonly used to denote an increase in the contact time between the vocal folds during a glottal cycle. This is mostly observed in patients with increased laryngeal muscle tension and those with reduced respiratory capacity [38, 39]. On the other hand, patients with hypoadduction of the vocal folds and a low subglottic pressure have flow phonation. The term breathy phonation is used to describe air leakage during phonation [40]. Common examples include patients with structural vocal fold disorders, bowing or atrophy of the vocal folds, and those with neurogenic voice disorders, such as vocal fold paresis or paralysis resulting in incomplete closure of the glottis [41]. Another determinant of loudness is the shape of the supraglottis. The supraglottis acts as a resonator that amplifies the vocal signal. Note that resonance, by definition, is "amplification of sound by a mechanism of reflection on various structures." As such, the reflection of the various harmonics on the supraglottic structures helps increase loudness.

The resonators and the formants: The resonators include structures that draw the boundaries of the airflow passage from the vocal folds to the lips, among which are the supraglottic structures, hypopharynx, oropharynx, nasopharynx, and oral cavity. Other components of the resonators are the nose and paranasal sinuses. The configuration and shape of the vocal tract determine the acoustic properties of the vocal signal and its harmonics. As such, the vocal tract acts as a filter that damps some frequencies and amplifies others. The formants are frequencies that fit best the resonators' qualities. They are primarily responsible for the speaker's voice timbre and attributes. Based on Johan Sundberg, F1 and F2 are mainly responsible for the vowel color, whereas F3, F4, and F5 relate to the personal voice timbre [42].

Given the intricate relationship between the shape of the vocal tract and sound, it stands to reason that one can tune his or her voice by narrowing, widening, lengthening, or shortening the vocal tract. This can be achieved by using the articulators such as the tongue, mandible, and lips. Protruding the lips or lowering the larynx can lower the formants, whereas shortening of the vocal tract can raise these formants. It is important to note that each formant is modulated preferentially by a given articulator. For instance, F1 is affected most by movement of the mandible, and F2 is mostly sensitive to the shape and position of the tongue. The third formant is determined primarily by the size of the oral cavity, and the fourth and fifth formants are very much dependent on the configuration of the lower pharynx and larynx [11]. The position and dispersion of the first four to five formants carry heavy implications for the quality of the singer's voice and his or her ability to sing louder. This is often referred to as Singer's formant, a peak prominence seen on a spectral envelope in the vicinity of 2300 Hz to 3200 Hz, which depends on the vocal register and loudness [43]. This peak prominence increases as we move from Bass to Baritone to Tenor, and increases with an increase in loudness. It is generated by clustering the energy and by reducing the interspace between the third, fourth, and fifth formants. This resonance is achieved by an articulatory phenomenon, namely widening the pharynx and lowering the larynx, allowing it to act as a separate resonator [44].

References

1. Sataloff RT. Clinical anatomy and physiology of the voice. In: Hamdan A-L, Sataloff RT, Hawkshaw MJ, editors. Obesity and voice. San Diego (CA): Plural Publishing; 2019. p. 33–81.
2. Chhetri DK, Jamal N. Percutaneous injection laryngoplasty. Laryngoscope. 2013;124(3):742.
3. Hately W, Evison G, Samuel E. The pattern of ossification in the laryngeal cartilages: a radiological study. Br J Radiol. 1965;38(452):585–91.
4. Randestad A, Lindholm CE, Fabian P. Dimensions of the cricoid cartilage and the trachea. Laryngoscope. 2000;110(11):1957–61.
5. Sataloff RT. Clinical anatomy and physiology of the voice. In: Sataloff RT, editor. Professional voice: the science and art of clinical care. 4th ed. San Diego (CA): Plural Publishing; 2017. p. 157–96.
6. Magaros NE. Anatomy of the vocal mechanism: structure of the voice. In: Benninger MS, Murray T, editors. The performer's voice. San Diego (CA): Plural Publishing; 2006. p. 15–22.
7. Woodson GE. Laryngeal and pharyngeal function. In: Flint PW, Haughey BH, Lund VJ, Niparko JK, Richardson MA, Robbins KT, Thomas JR, editors. Cummings otolaryngology: head and neck surgery. 5th ed. Philadelphia: Mosby Elsevier; 2010. p. 799–807.e1.
8. Toth J, Lappin SL. Anatomy, head and neck, mylohyoid muscle. 2023. In: StatPearls [Internet]. Treasure Island (FL): StatPearls Publishing; 2025. PMID: 31424877.
9. Rathee M, Jain P. Anatomy, head and neck, stylohyoid muscle. 2023. In: StatPearls [Internet]. Treasure Island (FL): StatPearls Publishing; 2025. PMID: 31613433.
10. Iwarsson J, Sundberg J. Effects of lung volume on vertical larynx position during phonation. J Voice. 1998;12(2):159–65.
11. Sundberg J. Vocal tract resonance. In: Sataloff RT, editor. Professional voice: the science and art of clinical care. 4th ed. San Diego (CA): Plural Publishing; 2017. p. 309–28.
12. Andaloro C, Sharma P, La Mantia I. Anatomy, head and neck: larynx arytenoid cartilage. 2023. In: StatPearls [Internet]. Treasure Island (FL): StatPearls Publishing; 2025. PMID: 30020624.
13. Ludlow CL. Laryngeal reflexes: physiology, technique, and clinical use. J Clin Neurophysiol. 2015;32(4):284–93. https://doi.org/10.1097/WNP.0000000000000187. PMID: 26241237; PMCID: PMC4527097.
14. Hoerter JE, Fakoya AO, Chandran SK. Anatomy, head and neck: laryngeal muscles. 2024. In: StatPearls [Internet]. Treasure Island (FL): StatPearls Publishing; 2025. PMID: 31424849.
15. Jurik AG, Pedersen U, Nøorgård A. Rheumatoid arthritis of the cricoarytenoid joints: a case of laryngeal obstruction due to acute and chronic joint changes. Laryngoscope. 1985;95(7 Pt 1):846–8.

16. Koch J, Unteregger F, Honegger F, Potthast S, Storck C. The cricothyroid joint: a practical guide for distinguishing between different joint types. J Voice. 2020;34(1):33–7.
17. Soriano RM, Winters R, Fakoya AO, Gupta V. Anatomy, head and neck: laryngeal nerves. 2024. In: StatPearls [Internet]. Treasure Island (FL): StatPearls Publishing; 2025. PMID: 32491674.
18. Maranillo E, León X, Quer M, Orús C, Sañudo JR. Is the external laryngeal nerve an exclusively motor nerve? The cricothyroid connection branch. Laryngoscope. 2003;113(3):525–9. https://doi.org/10.1097/00005537-200303000-00024. PMID: 12616208.
19. Suárez-Quintanilla J, Fernández Cabrera A, Sharma S. Anatomy, head and neck: larynx. 2023. In: StatPearls [Internet]. Treasure Island (FL): StatPearls Publishing; 2025. PMID: 30855790.
20. Sanders I, Mu L. Anatomy of the human internal superior laryngeal nerve. Anat Rec. 1998;252(4):646–56.
21. Ardito G, Revelli L, D'Alatri L, Lerro V, Guidi ML, Ardito F. Revisited anatomy of the recurrent laryngeal nerves. Am J Surg. 2004;187(2):249–53.
22. Sato K, Sato K. Blood vessels of the larynx and vocal fold. In: Functional histoanatomy of the human larynx; 2018. p. 287–303.
23. Levendoski EE, Leydon C, Thibeault SL. Vocal fold epithelial barrier in health and injury: a research review. J Speech Lang Hear Res. 2014;57(5):1679–91.
24. Verdolini K, Min Y, Titze IR, Lemke J, Brown K, Van Mersbergen M, Jiang J, Fisher K. Biological mechanisms underlying voice changes due to dehydration.
25. Alves M, Krueger E, Pillay B, Van Lierde K, Van der Linde J. The effect of hydration on voice quality in adults: a systematic review. J Voice. 2019;33(1):125–e13.
26. Zou ZF, Chen W, Li W, Yuan K. Impact of vocal fold dehydration on vocal function and its treatment. Curr Med Sci. 2019;39:310–6.
27. Franca MC, Simpson KO. Effects of hydration on voice acoustics. Contemp Issues Commun Sci Disord. 2009;36(Fall):142–8.
28. Hirano M, Kurita S, Nagata K. Layer structure of the vocal fold and its vibratory behavior. Jpn J Logoped Phoniatr. 1981;22(3):224–9.
29. Traser L, Burk F, Özen AC, Burdumy M, Bock M, Blaser D, Richter B, Echternach M. Respiratory kinematics and the regulation of subglottic pressure for phonation of pitch jumps—a dynamic MRI study. PLoS One. 2020;15(12):e0244539.
30. De Troyer A, Boriek AM. Mechanics of the respiratory muscles. Compr Physiol. 2011;1(3):1273–300.
31. Traser L, Özen AC, Burk F, Burdumy M, Bock M, Richter B, Echternach M. Respiratory dynamics in phonation and breathing—a real-time MRI study. Respir Physiol Neurobiol. 2017;236:69–77.
32. Aaen M, Sadolin C, McGlashan J. An integrative supraglottic sound source taxonomy (SSST) for pathological speaking voice: a case series. J Speech Lang Hear Res. 2025;68(5):2157–74.
33. Jiang J. Physiology of voice production: how does the voice work. In: Benninger MS, Murray T, editors. The performer's voice. San Diego (CA): Plural Publishing; 2006. p. 23–32.
34. Ghanem A, Hamdan AL. Unsedated office-based blue laser therapy in female patients with Reinke's edema: a retrospective review of 8 cases. J Voice. 2022;
35. Isshiki N, Ohkawa M, Goto M. Stiffness of the vocal cord in dysphonia—its assessment and treatment. Acta Otolaryngol. 1985;98(sup419):167–74.
36. Mastronikolis NS, Remacle M, Biagini M, Kiagiadaki D, Lawson G. Wendler glottoplasty: an effective pitch raising surgery in male-to-female transsexuals. J Voice. 2013;27(4):516–22.
37. Bozeman KW. Acoustic passaggio pedagogy for the male voice. Logoped Phoniatr Vocol. 2013;38(2):64–9. https://doi.org/10.3109/14015439.2012.679967. Epub 2012 Apr 19. PMID: 23763476.
38. Garaycochea O, Navarrete JM, Del Río B, Fernández S. Muscle tension dysphonia: which laryngoscopic features can we rely on for diagnosis? J Voice. 2019;33(5):812–e15.
39. Naqvi Y, Gupta V. Functional voice disorders. 2023. In: StatPearls [Internet]. Treasure Island (FL): StatPearls Publishing; 2025. PMID: 33085329.

40. Gordon M, Ladefoged P. Phonation types: a cross-linguistic overview. J Phon. 2001;29(4):383–406.
41. Marques JAS, Marronnier A, Crampon F, Lagier A, Marie JP. Early management of acute unilateral vocal fold paralysis: update of the literature. J Voice. 2021;35(6):924–6. https://doi.org/10.1016/j.jvoice.2020.02.021. Epub 2020 Apr 3. PMID: 32253078.
42. Sataloff RT. The physics of sound. In: Sataloff RT, editor. Professional voice: the science and art of clinical care. 4th ed. San Diego (CA): Plural Publishing; 2017. p. 91–102.
43. Bloothooft G, Plomp R. The sound level of the singer's formant in professional singing. J Acoust Soc Am. 1986;79(6):2028–33.
44. Rakerd B, Hunter EJ, Lapine P. Resonance effects and the vocalization of speech. Perspect ASHA Spec Interest Groups. 2019;4(6):1637–43.

4 Workup of Patients with Voice Disorders

This chapter provides an overview of the workup of patients presenting with hoarseness, with an emphasis on vocal history, auditory perceptual evaluation, and laryngeal examination. The use of the voice laboratory in the assessment of the dysphonic patient is also highlighted.

Patient History

Age and gender: Both gender and age must be considered in the workup of a patient with a voice disorder. Voice is an acoustic cue to our gender. Numerous studies indicate that the larynx is a hormonal target, and hormonal receptors for estrogen, progesterone, and testosterone have been identified in various laryngeal muscles and cartilages [1, 2]. As such, many voice disorders have been linked to fluctuations in sex hormones. Common examples include premenstrual vocal syndrome and postmenopausal vocal syndrome, which represent a constellation of symptoms including voice fatigue, throat clearing, and loss of the high notes [3, 4]. Voice is also an acoustic cue to our age. All three components of the phonatory apparatus change as we age. There is atrophy of the vocal folds' muscles and substantial alteration in the lamina propria constituents [5, 6]. Aging also leads to a decrease in respiratory capacity, the power source of phonation, and to changes in the shape and configuration of the resonators. The term "presbyphonia" is frequently used to describe the change in voice quality associated with aging.

Nature and onset of the voice complaint: The nature and onset of the voice complaint are often diagnostic clues in the workup of patients with voice disorders. Different terms are used by patients to describe the change in their voice quality. These include "hoarse voice," "raspy voice," "whispery voice," and "strangulated voice," among other terms. The term used by the patient may guide the physician toward the diagnosis and may be misleading. An acute onset is usually indicative of an abrupt vocal fold injury, such as bleeding or mucosal tear, whereas a chronic

A.-l. Hamdan, *E-Cigarette Smoking, Voice, and Health*, https://doi.org/10.1007/978-3-032-04913-1_4

onset is more indicative of an insidious disease, such as vocal fold nodules or a malignancy. It is important to note that voice symptoms are often associated with other laryngopharyngeal symptoms such as throat itching, oral dryness, globus sensation, and dysphagia. When these symptoms are present, confounding diseases such as allergy and reflux should be considered.

The impact of hoarseness on the patient's quality of life needs to be addressed as well in the workup of a dysphonia. It is a key determinant of any treatment plan. Several questionnaires have been described, such as the Voice Handicap Index noted by Jacobson et al. The VHI addresses the functional, physical, and emotional aspects of hoarseness, with higher scores being noted in patients with severe voice disorders [7]. A shorter version, the Voice Handicap Index-10, described by Rosen et al., has also been proven to have good reliability in assessing voice-related quality of life and in capturing patients' perceived voice impairment [8]. For the singing voice, Sataloff et al. described a more detailed questionnaire that covers other environmental and health risk factors [9].

Vocal hygiene and phonatory habits. The voice care provider needs to unveil any history suggestive of poor vocal hygiene. Common examples include a history of smoking and or insufficient intake of water. Note that dehydration can be systemic, secondary to fasting, vomiting and diarrhea, or local, secondary to mouth breathing or inhalation of dry desiccated air. Laryngeal desiccation may also be drug-induced following the intake of anticholinergics or the result of radiation therapy to the head and neck [5, 10–12]. Phonatory habits also play a paramount role in the etiology of voice disorders. Examples of bad phonatory habits include voice abuse, such as screaming and coughing, voice overuse, and misuse. An increase in the collision force between the vocal folds leads to an increase in the capillary pressure. In turn, this can result in leakage of fluid into the extracellular space, bleeding, fibrin deposition, and hyalinization.

Environmental risk factors: The physician should gather information on the patient's working environment. The inhalation of irritants and/or toxic substances may cause direct and indirect injury to the vocal folds. Allergy is a main culprit in patients with voice disorders. Patients with dysphonia are more likely to have an allergy than patients with no dysphonia, and patients with functional dysphonia are more likely to have an allergy than those with structural or neurologic voice disorders [13]. Looking at the other side of the coin, patients with allergy are also more prone to develop dysphonia than patients with no allergy [14–16]. This is in agreement with the unified airway concept by Krouse et al., which states that an allergy-induced inflammatory reaction at one site of the airway can result in a similar one at a different site of the airway. Noise is another environmental risk factor for hoarseness that warrants serious consideration in the workup of patients with voice disorders. Based on the World Health Organization (WHO), noise is a health risk factor associated with numerous morbidities, among which is dysphonia [17]. Background noise and poor acoustics, such as prolonged reverberation, can often lead to functional and structural voice disorders [18].

Systemic diseases. Because phonation is a complex motor and sensory process, a change in voice quality may often be the presenting symptom or one of the symptoms of a systemic disease. The laryngeal manifestations of the respiratory, endocrine, autoimmune, digestive, and neurologic systems are numerous. Voice care providers should be diligent in the system inquiry of patients with hoarseness, and should be alert to the adverse effects of systemic diseases on the phonatory apparatus. For instance, patients with diseases of the lower airway, such as chronic obstructive pulmonary disease (COPD) or asthma, are more likely to report voice symptoms secondary to a decrease in respiratory capacity or to the intake of steroid inhalers [19–23]. Gastrointestinal disorders can also markedly impact voice. The retrograde movement of the gastroduodenal contents to the larynx and pharynx may cause damage to the vocal folds and laryngeal mucosa, increasing the risk of benign and malignant lesions [24, 25]. Disorders of the neurologic system may also present with changes in voice quality and swallowing disorders. Patients with Parkinson's disease often present with voice fatigue, volume and pitch disturbance, and inability to control voice onset. These symptoms are attributed to poor laryngeal muscle control and hypo-adduction of the vocal folds during phonation. Similarly, patients with amyotrophic lateral sclerosis (ALS) can present with a decrease in voice intensity and aspiration secondary to dysfunction in the laryngeal and pharyngeal muscles [26]. Patients with essential tremor may complain of voice tremor with or without tremors of the extremities, an entity often referred to as "essential voice tremor" [27]. The laryngeal manifestations of autoimmune diseases are also numerous. Patients with rheumatoid arthritis can present with breathiness and aspiration as a result of unilateral vocal fold impaired mobility secondary to cricoarytenoid joint (CAJ) arthritis [28]. In the case of bilateral CAJ involvement, patients can present with stridor and difficulty in breathing [29]. Other rare causes of dysphonia in patients with autoimmune disorders include vocal fold Bamboo nodes. On laryngeal examination, Bamboo nodes present as unilateral or bilateral submucosal yellowish lesions transverse to the long axis of the vocal fold [30].

Medications: The effect of pharmacologic agents on voice has been extensively investigated in the literature. Medication-induced voice changes are primarily linked to the known mechanisms of action and/or the side effects of these medications. Biological variability and vocal hygiene play significant roles in modulating voice changes in response to medications. Therefore, it is essential to assess a patient's medication history when evaluating any change in voice quality [31]. The adverse effects of medications on voice have been investigated by numerous authors. In a systematic review on the influence of inhaled corticosteroid (ICS) on voice, Lechien et al. reported dysphonia in 34% of ICS users. The change in voice quality was associated with significant stroboscopic abnormalities and changes in acoustic parameters [32]. Haft et al. conducted a cross-sectional study on the association between anticholinergic medications and hoarseness in 149 patients. Medications examined included tramadol, bupropion, and alprazolam. Patients receiving two or more anticholinergic medications were 4.52 times more likely to experience dysphonia compared to those taking only one. A significant difference in the mean Voice Handicap Index-10 (VHI-10) score was observed between the two groups ($p = 0.023$) [33]. Thompson reviewed the impact of antihypertensive medications on voice, particularly diuretics, alpha adrenergic agonists, and angiotensin-converting enzyme inhibitors and noted vocal tract dryness and cough as major side effects [34]. Mattioni et al. highlighted the chemotherapy-induced side effects, such as diarrhea, nausea, and vomiting, which can cause transient dehydration, further compromising vocal quality [35]. Mattioni et al. also noted the neurotoxicity of some chemotherapeutic agents, such as vincristine, which can lead to vocal fold paralysis [35]. Hormonal therapy represents a pharmacologic class by itself, which can affect voice significantly [31]. Hamdan et al. investigated the effects of hormone replacement therapy (HRT) on voice in 53 menopausal women, 19 of whom were on HRT. While no significant difference in mean VHI-10 scores between those on HRT and those who were not noted, the former group had a significantly lower habitual pitch compared to the HRT group ($p = 0.022$), and women receiving HRT demonstrated significantly higher jitter ($p = 0.033$) [36]. The readers can refer to chapter 67 of the "Professional Voice: The Science and Art of Clinical Care," for more information on all medications that can affect the voice [37].

History of surgeries: Microlaryngeal surgery is a common cause of dysphonia. The change in voice quality is mostly due to inadvertent injury to the vocal ligament, which results in migration of collagen fibers to the Reinke space. This remodeling of the lamina propria landscape leads to a change in the viscoelastic properties of the vocal fold [38–40]. A change in voice quality may also be the result of alterations in vocal tract configuration. Common examples include cases following tonsillectomy, uvulopalatoplasty, and or surgical resection of oropharyngeal malignancies [41–43]. Similarly, patients undergoing orthodontic treatment such as rapid maxillary expansion should be alerted to the possible change in voice quality. The change in voice quality is attributed to an alteration in the position and dispersion of some of the formant frequencies.

Dysphonia is also a common complaint post-thyroidectomy and/or base of skull surgery. Injury to the recurrent laryngeal nerve is the most feared complication of thyroidectomy [44, 45]. The recurrent laryngeal nerve is also at risk in chest surgery, such as segmental lobectomy, mediastinoscopy, and open-heart surgery [46–48]. Abdominal surgery may also jeopardize the singing voice. Loss of abdominal support following hernia repair can be devastating to singers and professional voice users [9]. Last but not least, it is important to note that dysphonia can be an adverse complication of difficult intubation [49, 50]. Persistent dysphonia for more than 72 h after laryngeal manipulation should alert the physician to possible laryngeal trauma. Traumatic intubation in patients with a difficult airway and/or an anteriorly positioned larynx may lead to laryngeal/pharyngeal lacerations and vocal fold submucosal hemorrhage. Similarly, removal of the endotracheal tube cuff that is still inflated may result in a subluxation of the cricoarytenoid joint or injury to the vocal process [51, 52].

Auditory Perceptual Evaluation

Auditory perceptual evaluation is essential in the workup of a dysphonic patient. The perceived change in voice quality is often an acoustic cue to an underlying voice disorder. A raspy voice is suggestive of a vocal fold inflammation, whereas a breathy voice is indicative of a glottal insufficiency that can be secondary to a vocal fold paresis/paralysis, bowing, or scarring. A strained voice is suggestive of excessive laryngeal muscle tension, whereas a soft or whispery voice is suggestive of a psychogenic disorder. Decreased loudness and loss of intonation are suggestive of hypofunctional dysphonia or a depressive mood disorder. In rare instances, a volume disturbance may be a symptom of a decrease in hearing acuity, as phonation is a complex process that relies heavily on auditory feedback. Voice fatigue and worsening of voice quality toward the end of the day may be symptoms of a neurologic or neuromuscular disorder. Voice tremor is also a symptom suggestive of a central etiology and warrants a neurologic evaluation [53].

Different grading systems for dysphonia can be used to assist physicians in rating the severity of voice symptoms and their progress following therapy. The most commonly used system is the GRBAS scale, developed by "*The Japanese Society of Logopeadics and phoniatrics & The European Research Group*." In this scale, G stands for grade, representing the "overall degree of voice deviance"; R for roughness, referring to irregular fluctuations of the fundamental frequency (F0); B for breathiness, which reflects turbulent noise produced by air leakage; A for asthenia, indicating overall weakness of the voice; and S for strain, describing the impression of tension or effort during speech [54]. It is important to note that there are four important limitations to GRBAS: (i) inter-rater variability, (ii) examiner bias, (iii) lack of assessment of loudness, pitch, and timbre, and (iv) limited correlation with objective measures. Only three noise parameters correlate significantly with GRBAS: G correlates with VTI, NHR, and SPI; R correlates with NHR; A correlates with SPI; and B correlates with SPI [55].

Auditory perceptual evaluation of the singing voice is beyond the scope of this chapter. In addition to pitch, loudness, and timber, several other vocal characteristics are evaluated. These include resonance, intonation, or ability to hit the right note, vocal range, and presence or lack of vibrato, and the onset and offset of phonation, phrasing, and diction, among many other parameters. The reader can refer to chapter 79 of the "Professional Voice: The Science and Art of Clinical Care" [56].

Laryngeal Examination

Laryngeal examination starts with the palpation of the neck for any signs of stiffness, tenderness, or crepitation [53, 57]. A stiff or high-positioned larynx, narrowing of the thyrohyoid space, locking or fixed distance between the thyroid cartilage and cricoid, and point tenderness are signs of laryngeal muscle tension. Following examination of the neck, the larynx must be visualized to rule out structural or neurologic disorders. Viewing the larynx can be performed using a mirror, a flexible nasopharyngoscope, and/or a 70° or 90° telescope. Video-stroboscopic examination is also essential in the evaluation of the vibratory behavior of the vocal fold cover.

Flexible laryngoscopy: Laryngeal endoscopy using a flexible nasopharyngoscope is best performed without the use of a topical anesthetic to avoid drug-induced impairment in laryngeal sensation. Patient counselling before the introduction of the flexible nasopharyngoscope helps improve tolerance to the procedure [58]. The examination starts by introducing the flexible endoscope gently into the nasal cavity to the nasopharynx and hypopharynx. A narrow posterior airway space invariably denotes a sign of muscle tension. As the endoscope is introduced further down into the laryngeal inlet, the mucosal lining and contour of the larynx and pharynx are carefully examined for any lesions [59]. Pooling of mucus in the pyriform sinuses and impaired sensation should alert the physician to the possibility of a neurologic disease [60].

Flexible laryngoscopy allows the examiner to study the laryngeal posture and biomechanics, that is, the behavior of laryngeal structures in relation to time. By asking the patient to elicit sounds such as coughing, throat clearing, and laughing, the physician can assess the mobility of the vocal folds and glottal competence. The patient is also asked to perform the "ee-sniff" maneuver, which is extremely useful for the assessment of vocal fold mobility. In the case of a vocal fold paresis, the vocal fold lags following repetitive abduction and adduction [53, 61]. In addition, bowing of the vocal folds with incomplete closure of the vocal folds during phonation may also be seen in affected patients.

The supraglottic structures during phonation are also examined during flexible laryngoscopy. A laryngeal tilt and/or shortening of the aryepiglottic fold are signs suggestive of superior laryngeal nerve paralysis, while widening of the pyriform sinus and shortening of the vocal fold are signs often indicative of vocal cord paralysis. It is important to note that laryngeal asymmetry is not always pathologic, and arytenoid asymmetry may be a normal anatomic variant in many cases. Hirano et al., in their anatomical dissection of 50 larynges, documented a high prevalence of cricoid and thyroid cartilage asymmetry, particularly in the elderly [62]. The supraglottis is also examined for any signs of tension while the patient is asked to perform certain phonatory tasks. Common signs of laryngeal tension include medialization of the false vocal folds and or constriction of the distance between the petiole and inter-arytenoid surface [57]. Other signs of muscle tension dysphonia include incomplete closure of the vocal folds during phonation and false vocal fold vibration in extreme cases.

Telescopic examination; Telescopic examination of the larynx is usually performed using a 70° or 90° telescope. The good optical quality of a telescope allows the detection of any changes in color or texture of the mucosal lining of the laryngopharyngeal complex. This is extremely helpful in diagnosing inflammatory conditions such as laryngopharyngeal reflux disease. Telescopic examination is also of paramount importance in evaluating the vocal fold cover and in detecting mucosal lesions and submucosal lesions. Telescopic examination of the larynx is also useful in the evaluation of the supraglottic structures. A submucosal fullness often warrants further evaluation using computerized tomography and or magnetic resonance imaging of the larynx [63, 64].

Despite the added value of telescopic examination in terms of high optical quality and image magnification, there are many limitations to it; one is the need for patient tolerance. The presence of a strong gag reflex may prohibit the ability to introduce the telescope into the oropharynx [65]. A second limitation is the distorted position of the larynx when the patient is asked to protrude his or her tongue during examination [65]. A third limitation is the limited ability to study the laryngeal biomechanical behavior. The phonatory tasks required during telescopic examination are limited to the production of a sustained vowel and glissando. The physician cannot evaluate the larynx while the patient is asked to read a passage or sing. Another limitation is the limited angle of vision, particularly when using a 90° scope [66].

Laryngeal video-stroboscopy: The concept of stroboscopy was first introduced in cinematography [53, 57, 61]. It was later used for laryngeal examination in 1878. With the advances in technology and equipment, the use of stroboscopy has expanded over the years. Stroboscopy displays a montage of vocal fold vibration by summing multiple images of different glottal cycles [67]. Many methods in assessing stroboscopic examination have been proposed and standardized [61, 67–69], most common of which is SAMPC, described by M. Hirano [53, 67]. The "S" stands for symmetry, i.e., the extent to which one side mirrors the image of the opposite side; "A" stands for amplitude, which refers to the amount of lateral excursion of the vocal fold during phonation; "M" for mucosal wave, which begins at the lower lip of the vocal fold and travels toward the superior surface of the vocal fold; "P" for periodicity, which indicates that both vocal folds are vibrating in phase with each other or not; and "C" for closure of the vocal fold.

Laryngeal stroboscopic examination provides a wealth of information on the vibratory behavior and malleability of the vocal fold cover during phonation. This is extremely helpful in patients suspected of having vocal fold scars, sulcus vocalis, or fibrovascular masses. A decrease or absence of mucosal waves is a sign of vocal fold stiffness and alteration in the body-cover interface [70]. Stroboscopy is also useful in differentiating between the different pathologies of the vocal folds and in assessing glottic closure during phonation. Patients with structural voice disorders may exhibit incomplete vocal fold closure and a decrease in vocal fold mucosal waves at the site of the lesion during phonation. One example is bilateral vocal fold nodules, which often display an "hour-glass" opening on stroboscopic examination [71]. Hypo-adduction of the vocal folds and aperiodicity in vocal fold vibration are also signs commonly observed in patients with neuromuscular disorders such as Parkinson's disease [60].

Acoustic Analysis

Acoustic analysis provides an objective measure of vocal fold function that can be used to substantiate patient-reported outcome measures and auditory perceptual evaluation. It can also be used to monitor changes in voice quality following voice therapy, pharmacological treatment, and/or surgery. Various acoustic parameters can be extracted from a vocal signal, most common of which are fundamental frequency, cycle-to-cycle variations in frequency referred to as jitter, cycle-to-cycle variations in intensity referred to as shimmer, noise-to-harmonic ratio (NHR), voice turbulence index (VTI), and noise-to-harmonic ratio (NHR). The NHR measures the aperiodic noise in the vocal signal (best predictor of roughness) and the VTI measures the ratio of spectral inter-harmonic energy to spectral harmonic energy [72]. Other parameters include the Soft Phonation Index (SPI), which measures the average ratio of the lower frequency harmonic energy to the higher frequency.

It is important to note that acoustic analysis is not diagnostic of any specific voice disorder and hence has minimal specificity regarding a single vocal fold pathology. Another limitation of acoustic analysis is its restricted value in patients with severe hoarseness and in patients with an aperiodic vocal signal. When aperiodicity exceeds 5%, as in patients with a neurologic or neuromuscular disorder, acoustic measures should be interpreted cautiously [72].

Aerodynamic Measures

The most commonly used aerodynamic parameter in clinical practice is the maximum phonation time (MPT). It is measured by asking the subject to take a deep breath and phonate for as long as he or she can at a comfortable pitch and loudness. The test is usually repeated three times, and the higher value is considered for comparison with the norm. It is important to note that several factors may affect MPT. These include age, gender, number of trials, fatigability, and duration of apnea.

Another aerodynamic parameter that is also helpful in assessing glottis insufficiency is the mean flow rate (MFR). The mean flow rate or average phonation airflow varies with the type of phonation, the presence or absence of a vocal fold pathology, and the style of singing in singers. In patients with glottic insufficiency, the mean flow rate is increased because of incomplete closure of the vocal folds. The averaged or mean phonation air flow can be computed easily by dividing the vital capacity, defined as "the volume change at the mouth between the position of full inspiration and complete expiration," by the maximum phonation time [72, 73].

References

1. Newman SR, Butler J, Hammond EH, Gray SD. Preliminary report on hormone receptors in the human vocal fold. J Voice. 2000;14(1):72–81.

2. Hamdan AL, Sataloff RT, Hawkshaw MJ. Laryngeal manifestations of endocrine disorders. In: Hamdan AL, Sataloff RT, Hawkshaw MJ, editors. Laryngeal manifestations of systemic diseases. San Diego: Plural Publishing; 2019. p. 604–57.
3. Byeon H, Cha S. Evaluating the effects of smoking on the voice and subjective voice problems using a meta-analysis approach. Sci Rep. 2020;10(1):4720. https://doi.org/10.1038/s41598-020-61565-3. PMID: 32170174; PMCID: PMC7069957.
4. National Cancer Institute. Secondhand Tobacco Smoke (Environmental Tobacco Smoke) [Internet]. Bethesda (MD): National Cancer Institute; [cited 2025 May 9]. https://www.cancer.gov/about-cancer/causes-prevention/risk/substances/secondhand-smoke.
5. Hartley NA, Thibeault SL. Systemic hydration: relating science to clinical practice in vocal health. J Voice. 2014;28(5):652–e1.
6. Devadas D, More RS, Sahni C, Gupta M, Nayak AK, Mishra A. The aging larynx: an anatomical perspective. J Indian Acad Geriatr. 2022;18(4):221–6.
7. Jacobson BH, Johnson A, Grywalski C, Silbergleit A, Jacobson G, Benninger MS, Newman CW. The voice handicap index (VHI) development and validation. Am J Speech Lang Pathol. 1997;6(3):66–70.
8. Rosen CA, Lee AS, Osborne J, Zullo T, Murry T. Development and validation of the voice handicap index-10. Laryngoscope. 2004;114(9):1549–56. https://doi.org/10.1097/00005537-200409000-00009. PMID: 15475780.
9. Sataloff RT. Patient history. In: Sataloff RT, editor. Professional voice: the science and art of clinical care. 4th ed. San Diego, CA: Plural Publishing; 2017. p. 363–78.
10. Sivasankar M, Fisher KV. Oral breathing increases Pth and vocal effort by superficial drying of vocal fold mucosa. J Voice. 2002;16(2):172–81. https://doi.org/10.1016/s0892-1997(02)00087-5. PMID: 12150370.
11. Ito K, Izumi N, Funayama S, Nohno K, Katsura K, Kaneko N, Inoue M. Characteristics of medication-induced xerostomia and effect of treatment. PLoS One. 2023;18(1):e0280224.
12. Waghmare CM, Agarwal J, Bachher GK. Quality of voice after radiotherapy in early vocal cord cancer. Expert Rev Anticancer Ther. 2010;10(9):1381–8.
13. Hamdan AL, Abi Zeid Daou C, Karam M. Prevalence of allergy in patients with primary dysphonia. Indian J Otolaryngol Head Neck Surg. 2023;75(2):692–6. https://doi.org/10.1007/s12070-022-03403-8. Epub 2022 Dec 30. PMID: 37275010; PMCID: PMC10235223.
14. Randhawa PS, Nouraei S, Mansuri S, Rubin JS. Allergic laryngitis as a cause of dysphonia: a preliminary report. Logoped Phoniatr Vocol. 2010;35(4):169–74.
15. Simberg S, Sala E, Tuomainen J, Rönnemaa AM. Vocal symptoms and allergy—a pilot study. J Voice. 2009;23(1):136–9.
16. Turley R, Cohen SM, Becker A, Ebert CS Jr. Role of rhinitis in laryngitis: another dimension of the unified airway. Ann Otol Rhinol Laryngol. 2011;120(8):505–10.
17. World Health Organization. Guidelines for community noise. Berglund B, Lindvall T, Schwela DH, editors. Geneva: World Health Organization; 1999.
18. Cutiva LC, Burdorf A. Effects of noise and acoustics in schools on vocal health in teachers. Noise Health. 2015;17(74):17–22. https://doi.org/10.4103/1463-1741.149569. PMID: 25599754; PMCID: PMC4918643.
19. Tong JY, Sataloff RT. Respiratory function and voice: the role for airflow measures. J Voice. 2022;36(4):542–53.
20. Mohamed EE. Voice changes in patients with chronic obstructive pulmonary disease. Egypt J Chest Dis Tuberc. 2014;63(3):561–7.
21. Park B, Choi HG. Association between asthma and dysphonia: a population-based study. J Asthma. 2016;53(7):679–83.
22. Dogan M, Eryuksel E, Kocak I, Celikel T, Sehitoglu MA. Subjective and objective evaluation of voice quality in patients with asthma. J Voice. 2007;21(2):224–30.
23. Hamdan AL, Sataloff RT, Hawkshaw MJ. Laryngeal manifestations of respiratory disorders. In: Hamdan AL, Sataloff RT, Hawkshaw MJ, editors. Laryngeal manifestations of systemic diseases. San Diego: Plural Publishing; 2019. p. 306–45.

24. Lechien JR, Saussez S, Nacci A, Barillari MR, Rodriguez A, Le Bon SD, Crevier-Buchman L, Harmegnies B, Finck C, Akst LM. Association between laryngopharyngeal reflux and benign vocal folds lesions: a systematic review. Laryngoscope. 2019;129(9):E329–41.
25. Lu G, Ding X, Xu W. Association between laryngopharyngeal reflux and vocal fold leukoplakia. ORL. 2021;83(3):159–66.
26. Rautiola J, Laaksovirta H, Geneid A, Ilmarinen T, Pietarinen P, Kinnari TJ. ALS patients in otorhinolaryngology: a retrospective study. Laryngoscope Investig Otolaryngol. 2022;7(4):1071–7.
27. Sulica L, Louis ED. Clinical characteristics of essential voice tremor: a study of 34 cases. Laryngoscope. 2010;120(3):516–28.
28. Meng X, Xu HJ, Li RL, Zhao LD. Vocal cord lesions in representative autoimmune diseases. Clin Rheumatol. 2023;42(3):929–39. https://doi.org/10.1007/s10067-022-06411-9. Epub 2022 Oct 21. PMID: 36269532.
29. Kolman J, Morris I. Cricoarytenoid arthritis: a cause of acute upper airway obstruction in rheumatoid arthritis. Can J Anaesth. 2002;49(7):729–32. English, French. https://doi.org/10.1007/BF03017454. PMID: 12193494.
30. Hilgert E, Toleti B, Kruger K, Nejedlo I. Hoarseness due to bamboo nodes in patients with autoimmune diseases: a review of literature. J Voice. 2008;22(3):343–50. 51.
31. Sataloff RT, Hawkshaw MJ, Anticaglia J, White M, Meenan K, Romak JJ. Medications and the voice. In: Hamdan AL, Sataloff RT, Hawkshaw MJ, editors. Laryngeal manifestations of systemic diseases. San Diego: Plural Publishing; 2019. p. 663–717.
32. Lechien JR. Influence of inhaled corticosteroids on voice quality: a systematic review. J Voice. 2025;
33. Haft S, Farquhar D, Carey R, Mirza N. Anticholinergic use is a major risk factor for dysphonia. Ann Otol Rhinol Laryngol. 2015;124(10):797–802.
34. Thompson AR. Pharmacological agents with effects on voice. Am J Otolaryngol. 1995;16(1):12–8.
35. Mattioni J, Opperman DA, Solimando DA, Sataloff RT. Cancer chemotherapy: an overview and voice implications. J Sing. 2020;76(5):559–63.
36. Hamdan AL, Tabet G, Fakhri G, Sarieddine D, Btaiche R, Seoud M. Effect of hormonal replacement therapy on voice. J Voice. 2018;32(1):116–21.
37. Sataloff RT, Hawkshaw MJ, Anticaglia J, et al. Medications and the voice. In: Sataloff RT, editor. Professional voice: the science and art of clinical care. 4th ed. San Diego, CA: Plural Publishing; 2017. p. 1103–33.
38. Woo P, Casper J, Colton R, Brewer D. Diagnosis and treatment of persistent dysphonia after laryngeal surgery: a retrospective analysis of 62 patients. Laryngoscope. 1994;104(9):1084–91.
39. Benninger MS, Alessi D, Archer S, Bastian R, Ford C, Koufman J, Sataloff RT, Spiegel JR, Woo P. Vocal fold scarring: current concepts and management. Otolaryngol Head Neck Surg. 1996;115(5):474–82.
40. Svistushkin MV, Kotova S, Shpichka A, Starostina S, Shekhter A, Bikmulina P, Nikiforova A, Zolotova A, Royuk V, Kochetkov PA, Timashev S, Fomin V, Vosough M, Svistushkin V, Timashev P. Stem cell therapy for vocal fold regeneration after scarring: a review of experimental approaches. Stem Cell Res Ther. 2022;13(1):176.
41. Atan D, Apaydın E, Özcan KM, İkincioğulları A, Çetin MA, Dere H. Does tonsillectomy affect voice in early or late postoperative periods in adults? J Voice. 2017;31(1):131.e5–8. https://doi.org/10.1016/j.jvoice.2015.11.023. Epub 2016 Feb 1. PMID: 26846544.
42. Remade M, Betsch C, Lawson G, Jamart J, Eloy P. A new technique for laser-assisted uvulopalatoplasty: decision-tree analysis and results. Laryngoscope. 1999;109(5):763–8.
43. de Bruijn MJ, Rinkel RN, Cnossen IC, Witte BI, Langendijk JA, Leemans CR, Leeuw IM. Associations between voice quality and swallowing function in patients treated for oral or oropharyngeal cancer. Support Care Cancer. 2013;21:2025–32.
44. Cirocchi R, Arezzo A, D'Andrea V, Abraha I, Popivanov GI, Avenia N, Gerardi C, Henry BM, Randolph J, Barczyñski M. Intraoperative neuromonitoring versus visual nerve identification for prevention of recurrent laryngeal nerve injury in adults undergoing thyroid

surgery. Meta-analysis. Cochrane Database Syst Rev. 2019;1(1):CD012483. https://doi.org/10.1002/14651858.CD012483.pub2.
45. Henry BM, Vikse J, Graves MJ, Sanna S, Sanna B, Tomaszewska IM, Shane Tubbs R, Tomaszewski KA. Extralaryngeal branching of the recurrent laryngeal nerve: a meta-analysis of 28,387 nerves. Meta-analysis. Langenbeck's Arch Surg. 2016;401(7):913–23.
46. Cocuzza S, Di Luca M, Maniaci A, Russo M, Di Mauro P, Migliore M, Serra A, Spinato G. Precision treatment of post pneumonectomy unilateral laryngeal paralysis due to cancer. Future Oncol. 2020;16(16s):45–53.
47. Velez-Cubian FO, Toosi K, Glover J, Pancholy B, Hong E. Transient aphonia after mediastinoscopy. Case reports. Ann Thorac Surg. 2017;103(6):e549–50.
48. Hamdan A-L, Sibai A, Rameh C, Kanazeh G. Short-term effects of endotracheal intubation on voice. J Voice. 2007;21(6):762–8.
49. Sataloff RT. Cricoarytenoid and cricothyroid joint injury: evaluation and treatment. Treatm Voice Disord. 2005:289.
50. Brodsky MB, Akst LM, Jedlanek E, Pandian V, Blackford B, Price C, Cole G, Mendez-Tellez PA, Hillel AT, Best SR, Levy MJ. Laryngeal injury and upper airway symptoms after endotracheal intubation during surgery: a systematic review and meta-analysis. Meta-analysis. Anesth Analg. 2021;132(4):1023–32.
51. Chauhan A, Badhwar S, Patel M, Tiwari S. Post-intubation bilateral arytenoid dislocation with acute respiratory distress. J Anaesthesiol Clin Pharmacol. 2009;25(3):361–2.
52. Al Saeg AA, Alnori H. Laryngeal injury and dysphonia after endotracheal intubation. J Med Life. 2021;14(3):355.
53. Sataloff RT. Physical examination. In: Sataloff RT, editor. Professional voice: the science and art of clinical care. 4th ed. San Diego, CA: Plural Publishing; 2014. p. 391–403.
54. Yamaguchi H, Shrivastav R, Andrews ML, Niimi S. A comparison of voice quality ratings made by Japanese and American listeners using the GRBAS scale. Folia Phoniatr Logop. 2003;55(3):147–57.
55. Bhuta T, Patrick L, Garnett JD. Perceptual evaluation of voice quality and its correlation with acoustic measurements. J Voice. 2004;18(3):299–304. https://doi.org/10.1016/j.jvoice.2003.12.004. PMID: 15331102.
56. Baroody MM, Sataloff RT, Carroll LM. The singing voice specialist. In: Sataloff RT, editor. Professional voice: the science and art of clinical care. 4th ed. San Diego, CA: Plural Publishing; 2017. p. 1231–50.
57. Woo P. Laryngeal examinations and visualizations. In: Benninger MS, Murry T, editors. The performer's voice. 1st ed. San Diego: Plural Publishing; 2006. p. 73–89.
58. Paul BC, Chen S, Sridharan S, Fang Y, Amin MR, Branski RC. Diagnostic accuracy of history, laryngoscopy, and stroboscopy. Laryngoscope. 2013;123(1):215–9. https://doi.org/10.1002/lary.23630. Epub 2012 Oct 15. PMID: 23070976.
59. Sataloff RT, Hawkshaw M, Johnson JL, Ruel B, Wilhelm A, Lurie D. Prevalence of abnormal laryngeal findings in healthy singing teachers. J Voice. 2012;26(5):577–83.
60. Hamdan AL, Sataloff RT, Hawkshaw MJ. Laryngeal manifestations of neurologic disorders. In: Hamdan AL, Sataloff RT, Hawkshaw MJ, editors. Laryngeal manifestations of systemic diseases. San Diego: Plural Publishing; 2019. p. 171–229.
61. Woo P, Colton R, Casper J, Brewer D. Diagnostic value of stroboscopic examination in hoarse patients. J Voice. 1991;5(3):231–8.
62. Hirano M, Kurita S, Yukizane K, Hibi S. Asymmetry of the laryngeal framework: a morphologic study of cadaver larynges. Ann Otol Rhinol Laryngol. 1989;98(2):135–40.
63. Fang TJ, Lin WN, Lee LY, Young CK, Lee LA, Chang KP, et al. Classification of vocal fold leukoplakia by clinical scoring. Head Neck. 2016;38(1):E1998–2003.
64. Chen M, Li C, Yang Y, Cheng L, Wu H. A morphological classification for vocal fold leukoplakia. Braz J Otorhinolaryngol. 2019;85(5):588–96.
65. Hapner ER, Johns MM. Recognizing and understanding the limitations of laryngeal videostroboscopy. Perspect Voice Voice Disord. 2007;17(1):3–7.

66. Shao J, Stern J, Wang ZM, Hanson D, Jiang J. Clinical evaluation of 70 degrees and 90 degrees laryngeal telescopes. Arch Otolaryngol Head Neck Surg. 2002;128(8):941–4.
67. Hirano M. Phonosurgery: basic and clinical investigations. Otologia (Fukuoka). 1975;21:239–442.
68. Sataloff RT, Spiegel JR, Hawkshaw MJ. Strobovideolaryngoscopy: results and clinical value. Ann Otol Rhinol Laryngol. 1991;100:725–7.
69. Bless D, Hirano M, Feder RJ. Video stroboscopic evaluation of the larynx. Ear Nose Throat J. 1987;66:289–96.
70. Woo P. Objective measures of stroboscopy and high-speed video. Adv Otorhinolaryngol. 2020;85:25–44.
71. Dejonckere PH, Kob M. Pathogenesis of vocal fold nodules: new insights from a modelling approach. Folia Phoniatr Logop. 2009;61(3):171–9.
72. Dejonckere PH. Aerodynamic and acoustic voice measurements. In: Benninger MS, Murry T, editors. The performer's voice. 1st ed. San Diego: Plural Publishing; 2006. p. 90–102.
73. Jonathan RJ, Reinhardt JH, Hawkshaw M, Sataloff RT. The clinical voice laboratory. In: Sataloff RT, editor. Professional voice: the science and art of clinical care. 4th ed. San Diego, CA: Plural Publishing; 2014. p. 391–403.

Common Vocal Fold Pathology

5

There are numerous classifications for voice disorders based on etiology, auditory perceptual evaluation, and endoscopic findings. The most commonly adopted classification stratifies voice disorders into three categories: structural, neurologic, and functional. Patients are diagnosed with a structural voice disorder when a pathology is present on laryngeal endoscopy, such as a nodule, polyp, or cyst, and with a neurologic voice disorder when a laryngeal movement disorder, such as tremor, vocal fold paresis, or paralysis, is seen. In the absence of a structural and neurologic etiology, the patient is labeled as having a functional voice disorder.

In this chapter, the author discusses the most common vocal fold pathology encountered in otolaryngology practice. The objective is to provide the reader with an overview of structural voice disorders in patients presenting with hoarseness.

Laryngitis

Laryngitis is an inflammatory condition of the laryngeal tissues. The etiology is complex and includes trauma, infection, and systemic diseases [1]. Common examples include laryngopharyngeal reflux, allergy, and the inhalation of toxic substances such as smoke or other irritants [1]. The inflammatory cascade starts with dilatation of the vocal fold submucosal vessels and leakage of plasma fluid into the surrounding tissues, leading to edema and erythema. This is followed by infiltration of inflammatory cells and other chemical mediators, resulting in further damage. In the subacute form, fibrinous exudation as a by-product may be seen, whereas in the chronic form fibrosis and scaring may ensue as a result of enhanced activity of inflammatory cells and tissue destruction. The increase in cellular substrates, such as collagen, also contributes to the change in the viscoelastic properties of the vocal folds [2].

One of the most common causes of chronic laryngitis is smoking [1]. The persistent exposure of the laryngeal mucosa to the chemical irritants of smoke, namely tar,

A.-l. Hamdan, *E-Cigarette Smoking, Voice, and Health*,
https://doi.org/10.1007/978-3-032-04913-1_5

carbon monoxide gas, and nicotine particles, results in morphologic and physiologic changes. At the level of the vocal folds, there is attenuation of the fluidity of the vocal fold cover, resulting in dryness and an increase in friction between the vocal folds during phonation. This hygroscopic effect, secondary to inhaled pollutants, can precipitate mucosal injury and further the inflammatory response. In severe cases, laryngitis sicca may develop, leading to extensive erythema, swelling, and crust formation. Smoking may also precipitate phono-traumatic behavior such as cough and throat clearing as a result of excess mucus production and/or a change in its consistency [1]. In addition to hoarseness, patients may present with globus pharyngeus, sore throat, and odynophagia [1, 3]. The treatment of chronic laryngitis is focused primarily on voice hygiene therapy, such as cessation of smoking and proper hydration. The control of confounding factors such as reflux and allergy is also paramount. Vocal exercises to reduce laryngeal tension and improve voice production are also advocated [1, 3] (Fig. 5.1a, b).

Vocal fold nodules: Vocal fold nodules are benign exudative lesions of the lamina propria seen at the junction of the anterior and mid-third of the vocal folds, the site of maximum vibratory stress [4]. The lesions are more common in females with a history of voice overuse and or abuse. Affected patients often display strong extroversion traits in comparison to patients with other causes of hoarseness [5]. Another predisposing factor for the development of vocal fold nodules is reflux disease. Kuhn et al. reported a higher prevalence of laryngopharyngeal reflux in patients with vocal fold nodules compared to patients with normal vocal folds [6]. Using a 3-site pharyngoesophageal 24-h pH monitoring, Ulualp et al. reported pharyngeal acid reflux in 78% of patients with vocal fold nodules. The authors also noted a higher prevalence of posterior laryngitis in comparison to a control group [7]. Patients with vocal fold nodules often present with hoarseness, voice fatigue, and the need to exert effort to talk. In long-standing cases, patients may complain of neck pain and stiffness in the cervical muscles. On laryngeal examination, vocal

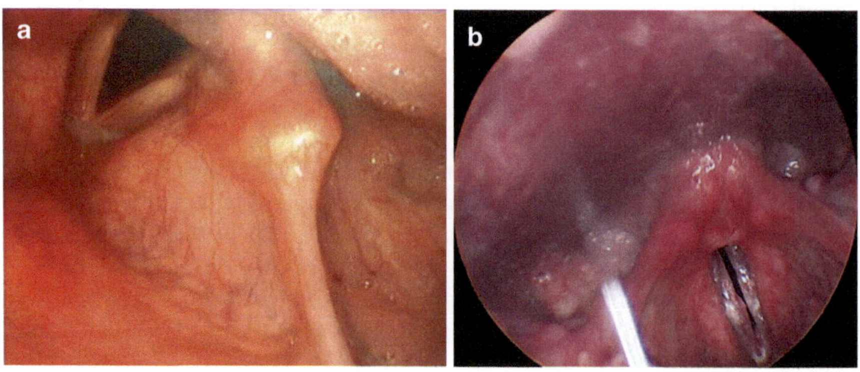

Fig. 5.1 (**a**) An endoscopic view of the larynx showing redness and edema of both vocal folds following an upper respiratory tract infection, suggestive of acute laryngitis. (**b**) An endoscopic view of the larynx showing severe inflammatory changes and irregularities of both vocal fold edges, suggestive of chronic laryngitis

fold nodules can be soft, fibro-edematous, or angio-ectatic depending on the duration of hoarseness and other confounding factors (Fig. 5.2a). Stroboscopy shows an hourglass opening during phonation, with or without impairment in the mucosal waves (Fig. 5.2b). The treatment of vocal fold nodules includes voice therapy and improvement in vocal hygiene. Other treatment modalities include office-based steroid injection under local anesthesia (Fig. 5.2c). In recalcitrant cases and patients with fibrous lesions, surgery may be recommended [8].

Vocal fold polyps: Vocal fold polyps are unilateral benign lesions of the vocal folds commonly encountered in men in their fourth and fifth decades [9]. Vocal history invariably reveals a history of phonotrauma. In a review of 784 patients with vocal fold polyps, Nagata et al. reported voice abuse as the most common etiologic factor [10]. Other risk factors include smoking and reflux disease. On laryngeal examination, polyps are mostly found at the anterior one-third of the vocal fold but may also be encountered anywhere along the membranous portion of the vocal fold. The lesion can be angiomatous, gelatinous, or with or without a reactive lesion on the contralateral vocal fold (Fig. 5.3a, b). Stroboscopy invariably shows a decrease in the mucosal waves and amplitude of vocal fold vibration at the site of the lesion.

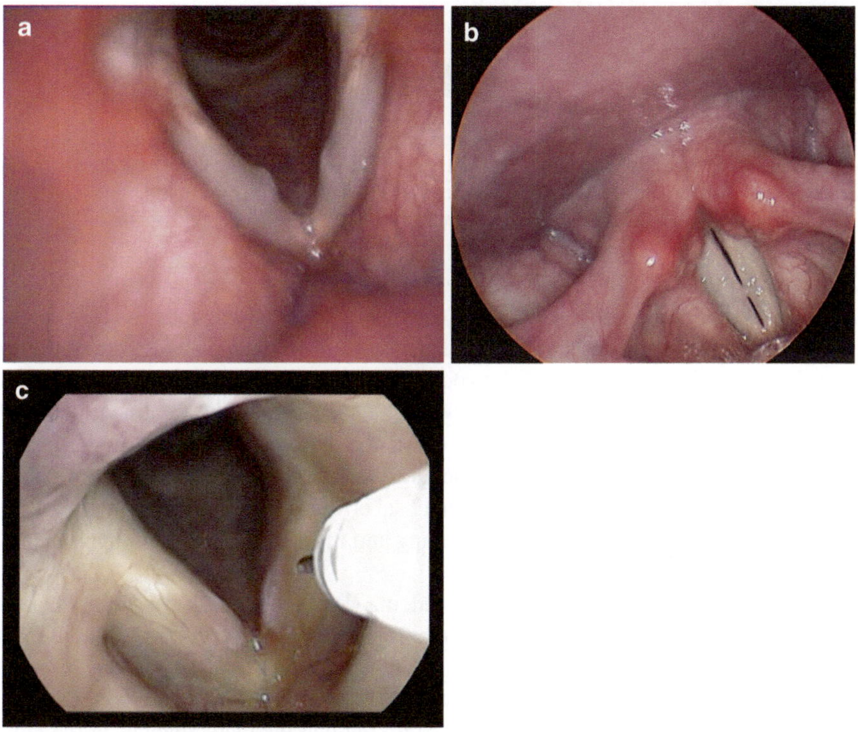

Fig. 5.2 (**a**) An endoscopic view of the larynx showing bilateral vocal fold nodules. (**b**) A stroboscopic view of the larynx showing an hourglass opening during phonation. (**c**) An endoscopic view of the larynx showing a 25-gauge flexible needle directed toward the left vocal fold fibro-edematous lesion for the injection of dexamethasone (8 mg/2 ml)

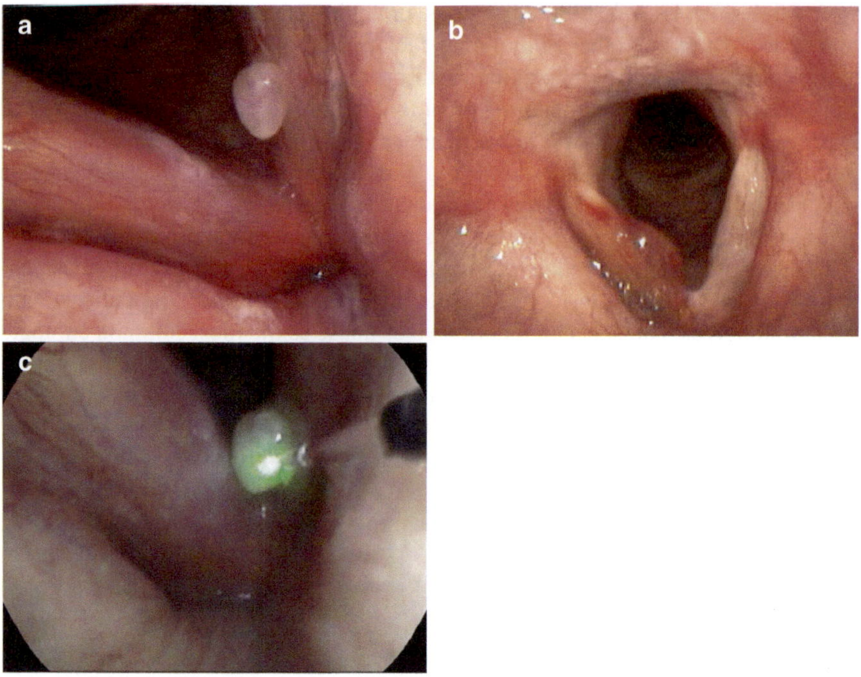

Fig. 5.3 (**a**) An endoscopic view of the larynx showing a left vocal fold gelatinous polyp. (**b**) An endoscopic view of the larynx showing a right vocal fold hemorrhagic polyp. Note the yellowish discoloration of the right vocal fold, suggestive of an old hemorrhage. (**c**) An intra-operative view showing the blue laser glass fiber (400 μm) directed toward the left vocal fold polyp

Incomplete closure of the vocal folds during phonation may be seen if the polyp is at the free edge of the vocal fold [11]. Co-existent vocal fold lesions, such as sulcus vocalis, are often seen on laryngeal endoscopy or during surgery [12]. In a review of 457 cases of benign lesions of the vocal folds, including polyps, Xiao et al. noted the presence of sulcus vocalis in 61.7% of the cases [13]. The treatment of vocal fold polyps is surgical in symptomatic patients. The surgery is traditionally performed in the operating room under general anesthesia. A microflap technique is commonly used to spare the overlying mucosal cover [14, 15]. Alternative treatment modalities include office-based laser therapy and intralesional steroid injection [16, 17] (Fig. 5.3c).

Vocal fold Reinke's edema: Reinke's edema (RE) is a benign condition characterized by the deposition of gelatinous material in the Reinke's space. Other terms such as diffuse corditis, polypoid degeneration, and polypoid laryngitis are often used to describe the same disease entity [18]. Women are more affected than men. The main risk factor for RE is smoking. Smoking can instigate changes in the lamina propria architecture and its extracellular matrix. Smoking may also result in mucosal changes such as hyperplasia and dysplasia. In a study that included 125 patients with RE, Marcotullio et al. noted an association between the rate of dysplasia and the duration of smoking [19]. Other precipitating factors for the development of RE include phono-trauma, reflux disease, and hypothyroidism. The retrograde movement of the gastroduodenal contents into the larynx results in mucosal and submucosal injury. Edema, ulceration, and granuloma formation may ensue following the exposure of the laryngeal mucosal lining to the acidic and non-acidic refluxate. Laryngopharyngeal reflux may also weaken the vocal fold defense mechanism by increasing cell-to-cell dehiscence [20].

Patients with RE present with deepening of the voice and loss of power. Other voice complaints include voice fatigue and the inability to project the voice. On laryngeal examination, there is an outpouching of the vocal fold, which can be unilateral or bilateral (Fig. 5.4a). The severity of the disease can be graded using various grading systems based on the extent of involvement of the vocal fold and impingement of the lesion on the glottic aperture [21, 22]. Notably, patients with advanced disease can present with symptoms of airway obstruction, dyspnea, and obstructive sleep apnea [23]. Hamdan et al. reported an association between disease severity and obstructive sleep apnea [23]. On stroboscopic examination, there is asymmetry, aperiodicity, and alteration in mucosal waves during phonation [24]. The first line of treatment for RE is vocal hygiene therapy and cessation of smoking. Control of confounding factors such as reflux disease is paramount. In patients who fail voice therapy, office-based intralesional steroid injection or laser therapy is

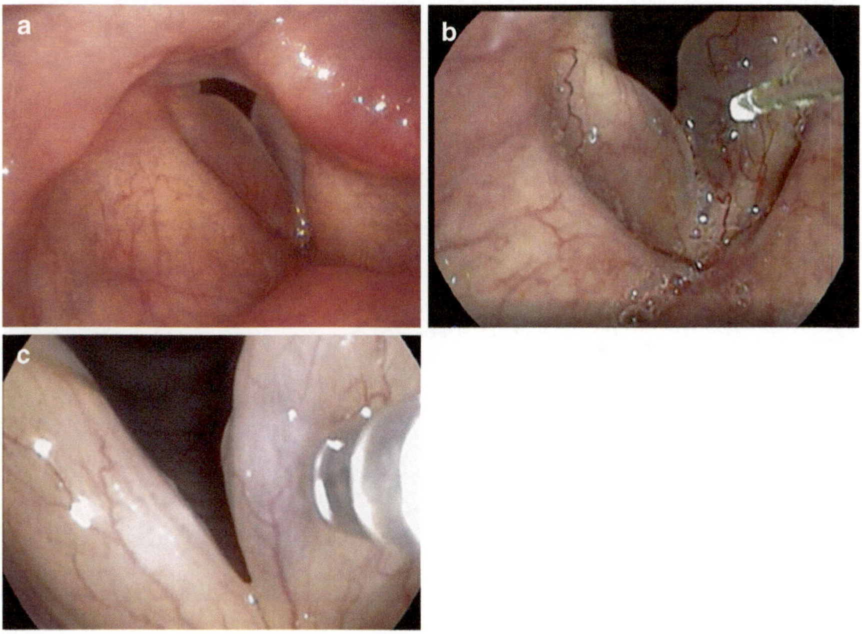

Fig. 5.4 (**a**) An endoscopic view of the larynx showing bilateral vocal fold Reinke's edema. (**b**) An intra-operative view of the larynx showing the blue laser glass fiber (400 µm) aiming at the Reinke's edema of the left vocal fold. (**c**) An endoscopic view of the larynx showing injection of dexamethasone (8 mg/2 ml) into the left vocal fold Reinke's edema using a 25-gauge flexible needle

advocated [17, 25–27] (Fig. 5.4b, c). Injection of other pharmaceutical agents, such as hyaluronidase, is also effective in many cases [28]. In severe cases refractory to conservative treatment, surgery may be recommended.

Vocal fold cysts: Vocal fold cysts are benign lesions of the vocal folds. These are stratified into epithelial inclusion cysts and mucus retention cysts. Epithelial cysts result from submucosal entrapment of epithelial remnants, whereas mucus retention cysts arise from obstruction of mucus glands. Poor vocal hygiene and phono-trauma are the main precipitating factors. Although vocal fold cysts may be found accidentally on laryngeal examination, affected patients invariably present with a change in voice quality. Voice complaints include hoarseness, voice fatigue, voice breaks, and diplophonia. On laryngeal examination, a vocal fold mucus retention cyst looks like a yellowish submucosal mass, whereas an epithelial inclusion cyst has a white pearl appearance (Fig. 5.5a, b). A decrease in mucosal waves and asymmetry with incomplete closure of the vocal folds are common findings on stroboscopic examination

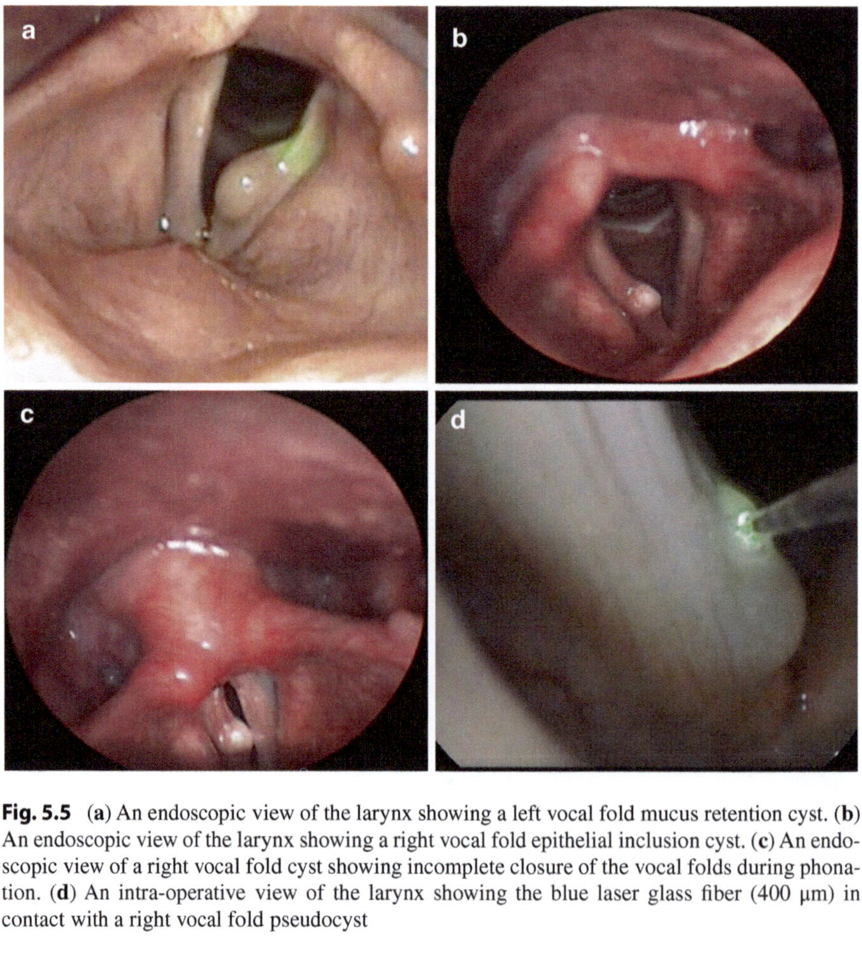

Fig. 5.5 (**a**) An endoscopic view of the larynx showing a left vocal fold mucus retention cyst. (**b**) An endoscopic view of the larynx showing a right vocal fold epithelial inclusion cyst. (**c**) An endoscopic view of a right vocal fold cyst showing incomplete closure of the vocal folds during phonation. (**d**) An intra-operative view of the larynx showing the blue laser glass fiber (400 μm) in contact with a right vocal fold pseudocyst

(Fig. 5.5c). The treatment of vocal fold cysts is surgical, although intralesional steroid injection has been advocated by some authors [26]. During microlaryngeal surgery, a mucosal flap is raised and the cyst is excised in total using cold steel instruments and or lasers [29]. An alternative treatment is marsupialization, which consists of removing part of the wall of the cyst to allow extrusion of its contents [30] (Fig. 5.5d).

Varices and ectasias: The vocal fold microvasculature has a distinctive pattern and histologic features. The submucosal vessels run along the long axis of the vocal folds and have an abundance of arteriovenous anastomoses. These features contribute to the enhanced malleability of the vocal fold cover and its durability in sustaining the mechanical stress of phonation [31]. Despite the sophistication of the vocal fold microvasculature, aberrant patterns are frequently encountered in otolaryngology practice. The most commonly observed ones are dilated vessels referred to as varices, and aggregations or coalescences of different vessels referred to as ectasias [31, 32]. These aberrations are more frequently encountered in women and in subjects with a high vocal load. The fluctuation in sex hormones and the increase in phonatory stress are the main precipitating factors for the development of these lesions. Another risk factor is the intake of anticoagulants. The clinical significance of ectasias and varices is still an issue of investigation among voice care providers. Affected patients may be asymptomatic or may present with a constellation of vocal symptoms [33]. These include hoarseness, voice fatigue, and inability to project the voice. Singers may complain of a contracted vocal range, loss of the high notes, and difficulty in transition between vocal registers. On laryngeal examination, vocal fold varices and ectasias are mostly seen at the upper surface of the vocal folds, and in the area of maximum phonatory stress referred to as the "striking zone" (Figs 5.6a, b). On stroboscopic examination, a decrease in mucosal waves at the site of the lesion may be seen. Another commonly observed endoscopic finding is a yellowish discoloration of the vocal fold. This latter is ascribed to hemosiderin deposition following submucosal hemorrhage [31]. The treatment of vocal fold varices and ectasias is advocated in symptomatic patients and in cases of recurrent vocal fold hemorrhage. Office-based laser therapy is highly efficacious (Fig. 5.6c, d).

Vocal fold scars: Vocal fold scars are a common cause of dysphonia. The most frequent etiology is injury to the vocal ligament during microlaryngeal surgery. Other causes include autoimmune and infectious diseases. Vocal fold scarring is characterized by a change in the extracellular matrix constituents of the lamina propria with deposition of collagen fibers in the superficial layer of the lamina propria. There are various degrees of vocal fold scarring based on the extent of involvement of the different layers of the lamina propria and vocalis muscle [34]. Affected patients can present with a change in pitch, disturbance in volume, and voice fatigue. Acoustic and aerodynamic analyses invariably show an increase in the perturbation parameters and a decrease in the mean flow rate in the case of glottic insufficiency. On stroboscopy, there is a decrease or absence of mucosal waves with phase asymmetry at the site of the scar (Fig. 5.7a). Bowing of the vocal folds and incomplete closure may be seen in patients with vocal fold soft tissue defects. A multidisciplinary approach is needed to treat vocal fold scars. Voice therapy aims at improving

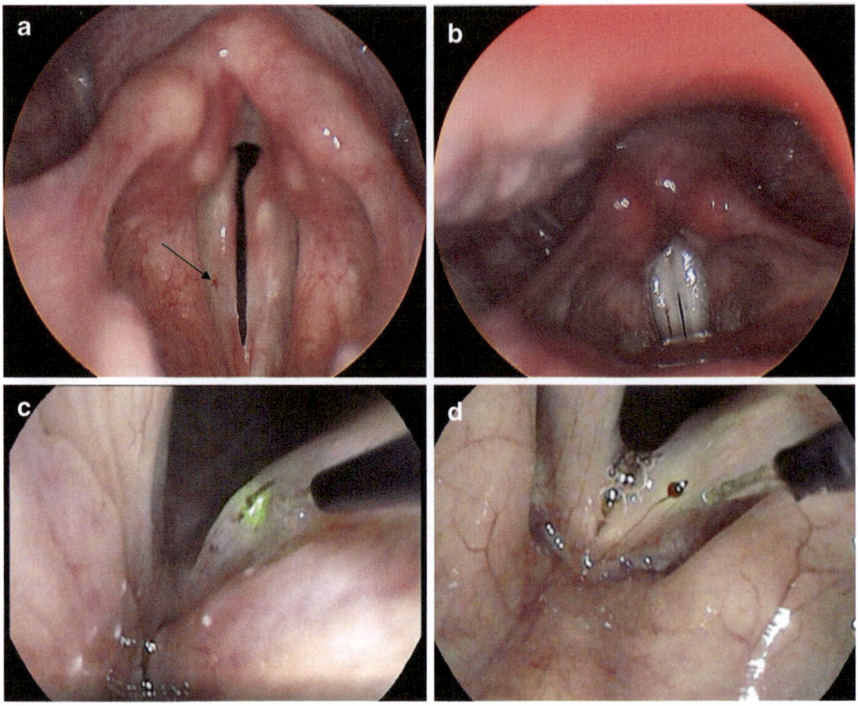

Fig. 5.6 (**a**) An endoscopic view of the larynx showing a left vocal ectasia. (**b**) An endoscopic view of the larynx showing a right vocal fold dilated vessel. (**c**) Intra-operative view of the larynx showing the blue laser glass fiber (400 μm) targeting the dilated vessel in non-contact mode. (**d**) Intra-operative view of the larynx showing the blue laser glass fiber (400 μm) targeting a left vocal fold hemorrhagic lesion in non-contact mode

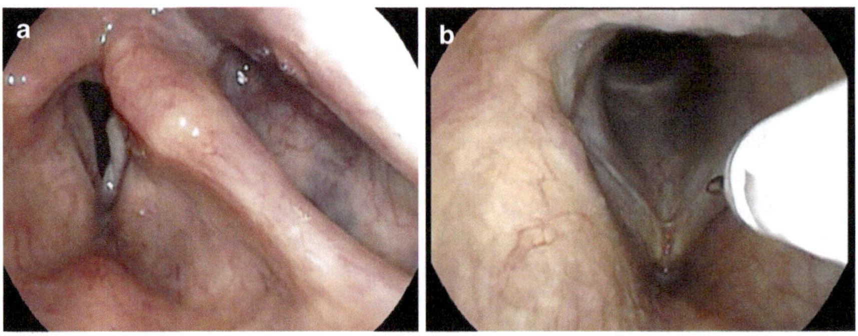

Fig. 5.7 (**a**) An endoscopic view of the larynx showing incomplete closure of the vocal folds during phonation secondary to a left vocal fold scar following microlaryngeal surgery. (**b**) An endoscopic view of the larynx showing a 25-gauge flexible needle directed toward the scar on the right vocal fold

the malleability of the vocal fold cover and enhancing voice production. Different surgical techniques have been described, including excision of the scar with or without the interposition of a graft between the mucosal cover and the underlying structures. Other treatment options include injection of steroids and laser therapy. Regenerative medicine using platelet-rich plasma, fibroblast growth factors, and stem cell therapy is on the rise (Fig. 5.7b).

Vocal fold leukoplakia: Vocal fold leukoplakia is characterized by whitish discoloration of the vocal fold mucosa. As the mucosal lining of the vocal fold is non-keratinizing, the presence of a whitish discoloration invariably underscores an underlying pathologic transformation. The consensus is that half of these lesions are inflammatory in origin, while the other half contain dysplastic or malignant cells. Based on the World Health Organization (WHO) classification, dysplastic lesions can be stratified as low-grade with no cellular atypia or high-grade with changes suggestive of mitosis and atypical cellular atypia [35, 36]. Isenberg et al. reviewed more than 200 cases and noted the presence of severe dysplasia and/or carcinoma in situ in almost one out of seven patients. Despite the relatively low prevalence of carcinoma in vocal fold leukoplakia, it is important to note that even inflammatory lesions and those with low-grade dysplasia may undergo malignant transformation in the long term [37]. The main risk factors for vocal fold leukoplakia are smoking and reflux disease. Numerous studies suggested a positive correlation between duration and extent of smoking and malignant transformation [38]. This is not surprising given that more than two-thirds of patients presenting with vocal fold leukoplakia are current or former smokers [38]. Reflux disease also plays an etiologic role in the development of these lesions. Many authors have documented abnormal 24-h pH-metry and alterations in esophageal impedance in patients with pre-malignant and malignant lesions of the vocal folds.

Patients with vocal fold leukoplakia invariably present with a change in voice quality. The voice is often described as harsh or breathy, particularly when the lesion is at the free edge of the vocal fold. When the lesion is on the upper surface of the vocal fold, patients may be asymptomatic. On laryngeal examination, the lesion may involve part or the entire surface of the vocal fold. It can be flat or elevated, smooth or rough, with regular or irregular edges (Fig. 5.8a). Many authors investigated the clinical significance of the lesion morphology. A large and elevated lesion with a rough surface is more likely to harbor dysplastic and malignant cells in comparison to a small, flat, and smooth lesion [39]. Stroboscopic examination also has a predictive value. A decrease in mucosal waves and incomplete closure of the vocal folds are ominous signs. An impairment in the mucosal waves has been noted in almost one-fourth of patients with dysplastic lesions and one-half of those with malignancy [40–42]. Narrow-band imaging is also useful in differentiating between malignant and non-malignant lesions and in predicting malignant transformation. Common findings include neovascularization and aberrant vascular patterns adjacent to the lesion [43]. Vocal fold leukoplakia warrants a tissue diagnosis. The biopsy can be done in the operating room or in the office. Office-based laryngeal biopsy has been shown to be efficacious with a high diagnostic yield (Fig. 5.8b). The treatment of vocal fold leukoplakia is multifaceted. Nonsuspicious lesions may be observed closely and managed with vocal hygiene therapy. Suspicious lesions

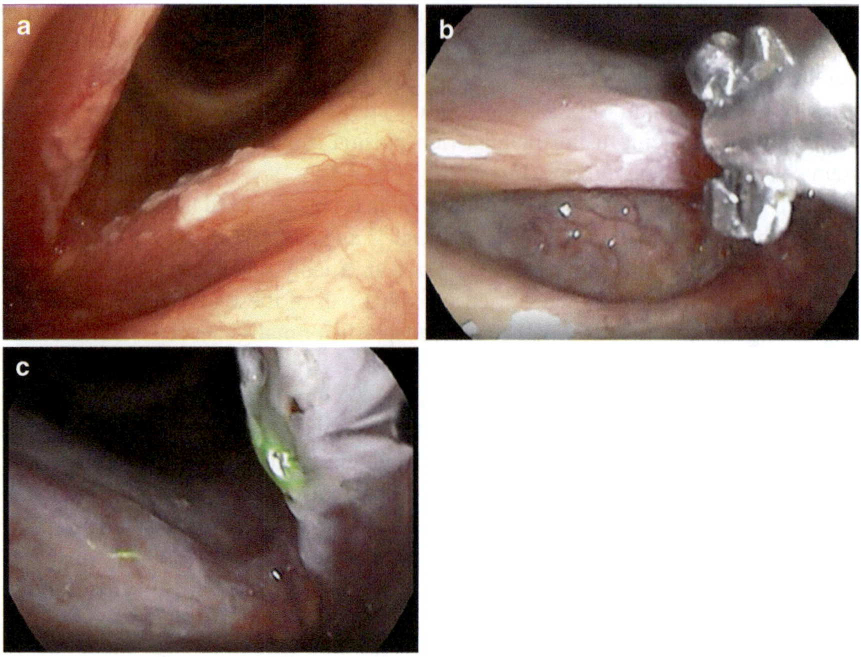

Fig. 5.8 (**a**) An endoscopic view of the larynx showing hyperkeratosis of both vocal folds. (**b**) An endoscopic view of the larynx showing the cup forceps directed toward a right vocal fold leukoplakia. (**c**) Intra-operative view of the larynx showing the blue laser glass fiber in contact with the left vocal fold leukoplakia

can be surgically removed or treated with lasers (Fig. 5.8c). In the presence of a malignancy, various types of cordectomy or radiation therapy are recommended.

Laryngeal recurrent respiratory papillomatosis: Recurrent respiratory papillomatosis (RRP) is a feared laryngeal pathology given its high rate of recurrence and long-term morbidity. The most common etiology is human papillomavirus. More than 200 strains have been identified, with the most common being HPV 6 and 11 [44]. Recurrent respiratory papillomatosis can affect any age but is mostly seen in the pediatric age group and adults. In the pediatric age group, the disease may be transmitted perinatally or by hetero-inoculation [45]. In adults, RRP is a sexually transmitted disease with a higher prevalence being noted in patients with multiple sexual partners. Other risk factors include infection with the herpes simplex type. Formanek et al. reported herpes simplex type 2 in 45% of the cases in a cohort of 40 patients [45].

The clinical presentation of RRP varies. Although it is often an incidental finding on laryngeal examination, affected patients can present with a myriad of symptoms related to voice and swallowing. The most commonly reported symptoms include hoarseness, foreign body sensation, dysphagia, and dyspnea. In severe cases, symptoms of upper airway obstruction, such as stridor, may prevail. On laryngeal examination, RRP has a distinctive cauliflower appearance. The lesion can be found anywhere on the mucosal surface of the laryngopharyngeal complex but is mostly seen at the squamous-columnar mucosal junction [46] (Fig. 5.9a). Narrow band imaging highlights the vascularity of the lesion and hence improves diagnosis [47].

Treatment of RRP is surgical. With the reform in laryngeal practice and the shift from the operating room to the clinic, many patients are treated in-office under local anesthesia. The use of photoangiolytic lasers has enhanced disease regression and decreased the risk of vocal fold scarring (Fig. 5.9b). Adjunct therapy using pharmaceutical agents has reduced the need for surgical intervention and has prolonged disease-free intervals.

Laryngeal cancer: Laryngeal cancers are among the most common malignancies of the head and neck, accounting for almost 1% of all cancers worldwide [48]. The most common risk factors are smoking and excessive alcohol intake. Numerous studies have shown that smokers are at a higher risk of having laryngeal cancer than non-smokers. Other predisposing factors include reflux disease, occupational exposure to inhaled toxic substances, and human papilloma virus infection [49]. Squamous cell carcinoma is the most common form of laryngeal cancer, accounting for almost 90% of all laryngeal malignancies. The glottis is affected in 60% of cases (Fig. 5.10). Given its location, patients are more likely to seek medical attention and hence be diagnosed early. For early-stage laryngeal cancer, patients are treated either surgically or by radiation. The transoral approach is commonly used under general anesthesia. Both diode and photoangiolytic lasers have been used for tumor resection, with good local control and laryngeal preservation [50]. In a systematic review on transoral laser microsurgery vs. radiotherapy for early glottic cancer, Vasudevan et al. reported superior results using the transoral surgery for patients with anterior commissure involvement [51]. In advanced cases, partial or total laryngectomy may be performed. Alternatively, chemoradiation may be advocated for organ preservation [52].

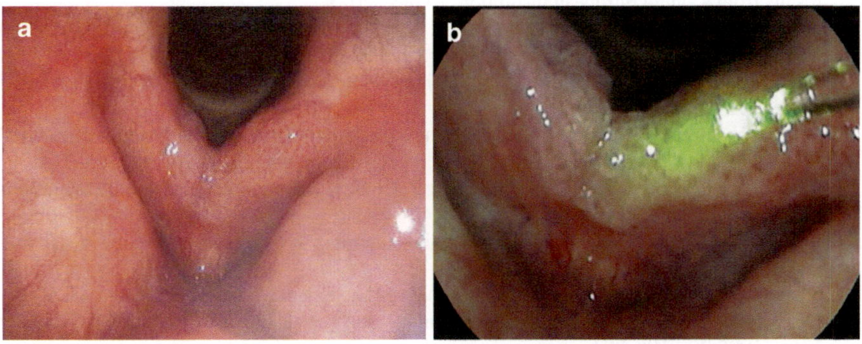

Fig. 5.9 (**a**) An endoscopic view of the larynx showing a recurrent respiratory papillomatous lesion. (**b**) Intra-operative view of the larynx showing the blue laser glass fiber directed toward the lesion

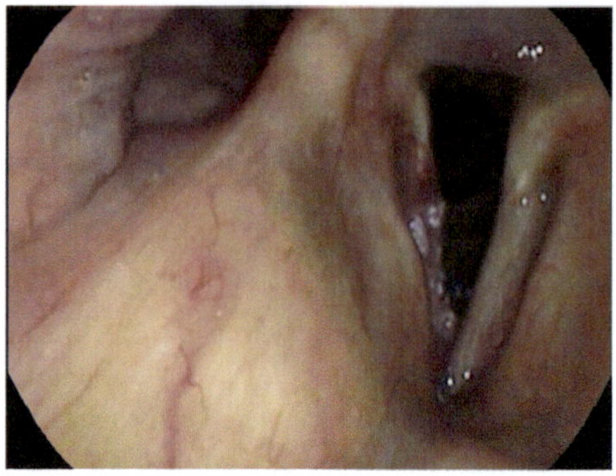

Fig. 5.10 An endoscopic view of the larynx showing a right vocal fold squamous cell carcinoma

References

1. Jetté M. Toward an understanding of the pathophysiology of chronic laryngitis. Perspect ASHA Spec Interest Groups. 2016;1(3):14–25. https://doi.org/10.1044/persp1.sig3.14. Epub 2016 Mar 1. PMID: 32864454; PMCID: PMC7451247.
2. Dworkin JP. Laryngitis: types, causes, and treatments. Otolaryngol Clin N Am. 2008;41(2):419–36.
3. Stein DJ, Noordzij JP. Incidence of chronic laryngitis. Ann Otol Rhinol Laryngol. 2013;122(12):771–4. https://doi.org/10.1177/000348941312201207. PMID: 24592580.
4. Titze IR. Mechanical stress in phonation. J Voice. 1994;8(2):99–105.
5. Roy N, Bless DM, Heisey D. Personality and voice disorders: a multitrait-multidisorder analysis. J Voice. 2000;14(4):521–48.
6. Kuhn J, Toohill RJ, Ulualp SO, Kulpa J, Hofmann C, Arndorfer R, Shaker R. Pharyngeal acid reflux events in patients with vocal cord nodules. Laryngoscope. 1998;108(8):1146–9.
7. Ulualp SO, Toohill RJ, Shaker R. Pharyngeal acid reflux in patients with single and multiple otolaryngologic disorders. Otolaryngol Head Neck Surg. 1999;121(6):725–30.
8. Murry T, Woodson GE. A comparison of three methods for the management of vocal fold nodules. J Voice. 1992;6(3):271–6.
9. Brunner E, Eberhard K, Gugatschka M. Prevalence of benign vocal fold lesions: long-term results from a single European institution. J Voice. 2023.
10. Nagata K, Kurita S, Yasumoto S, Maeda T, Kawasaki H, Hirano M. Vocal fold polyps and nodules. A 10-year review of 1,156 patients. Auris Nasus Larynx. 1983;10:S27–35.
11. Kenny HL, Friedman L, Simpson CB, McGarey PO. Vocal fold polyps: a scoping review. J Voice. 2023.
12. Sünter AV, Kırgezen T, Yiğit Ö, Çakır M. The association of sulcus vocalis and benign vocal cord lesions: intraoperative findings. Eur Arch Otorrinolaringol. 2019;276(11):3165–71.
13. Xiao Y, Liu F, Ma L, Wang T, Guo W, Wang J. Clinical analysis of benign vocal fold lesions with occult sulcus vocalis. J Voice. 2019;35(4):646–50.
14. Courey MS, Garrett CG, Ossoff RH. Medial microflap for excision of benign vocal fold lesions. Laryngoscope. 1997;107(3):340–4.
15. Sataloff RT, Spiegel JR, Heuer RJ, Baroody MM, Emerich KA, Hawkshaw MJ, Rosen DC. Laryngeal mini-microflap: a new technique and reassessment of the microflap saga. J Voice. 1995;9(2):198–204.
16. Hamdan AL, Hosri J, Feghali PAR, Abi Zeid Daou C, Ghanem A. Office-based blue laser therapy of vocal fold polyps: a cohort of 18 patients: blue laser therapy of vocal fold polyps. Laryngoscope. 2023;133(10):2712–8. https://doi.org/10.1002/lary.30602. Epub 2023 Feb 8. PMID: 36752582.
17. Hamdan AL, Hosri J, Daou CAZ, Ghzayel L, Hadi J, Saab MB, Kasti M, Mourad M. Office-based steroid injection for benign lesions of the vocal folds: case series and review of the lit-

erature. J Voice. 2024:S0892-1997(24)00095-X. https://doi.org/10.1016/j.jvoice.2024.03.023. PMID: 38762397.
18. Druck Sant'Anna G, Mauri M. Use of the microdebrider for Reinke's edema surgery. Laryngoscope. 2000;110(12):2114–6.
19. Marcotullio D, Magliulo G, Pezone T. Reinke's edema and risk factors: clinical and histopathologic aspects. Am J Otolaryngol. 2002;23(2):81–4.
20. Lechien JR, Saussez S, Nacci A, et al. Association between laryngopharyngeal reflux and benign vocal folds lesions: a systematic review. Laryngoscope. 2019;129(9):E329–41.
21. Tan M, Bryson PC, Pitts C, Woo P, Benninger MS. Clinical grading of Reinke's edema. Laryngoscope. 2017;127(10):2310–3. https://doi.org/10.1002/lary.26647. Epub 2017 Jun 5. PMID: 28581063.
22. Tavaluc R, Herman H, Lin J, Tan M. Does Reinke's edema grade determine premalignant potential? Ann Otol Rhinol Laryngol. 2018;127(11):812–6. https://doi.org/10.1177/0003489418796529. Epub 2018 Sep 6. PMID: 30187764.
23. Hamdan AL, Khalifee E, Abi Akl PR, Ghanem A, El Hage A. Pathogenic role of Reinke's edema in snoring and obstructive sleep apnea. J Voice. 2020;34(3):456–9. https://doi.org/10.1016/j.jvoice.2018.12.001. Epub 2018 Dec 15. PMID: 30563731.
24. Tavaluc R, Tan-Geller M. Reinke's edema. Otolaryngol Clin N Am. 2019;52(4):627–35.
25. Ghanem A, Hamdan AL. Unsedated office-based blue laser therapy in female patients with Reinke's edema: a retrospective review of 8 cases. J Voice. 2025;39(2):525–30. https://doi.org/10.1016/j.jvoice.2022.08.025. Epub 2022 Oct 9. PMID: 36220740.
26. Wang CT, Liao LJ, Cheng PW, Lo WC, Lai MS. Intralesional steroid injection for benign vocal fold disorders: a systematic review and meta-analysis. Laryngoscope. 2013;123(1):197–203. https://doi.org/10.1002/lary.23551. Epub 2012 Sep 10. PMID: 22965481.
27. Lee SW, Park KN. Long-term efficacy of percutaneous steroid injection for treating benign vocal fold lesions: a prospective study. Laryngoscope. 2016;126(10):2315–9. https://doi.org/10.1002/lary.25916. Epub 2016 Mar 12. PMID: 26971530.
28. Woo P. Hyaluronidase injection in the vocal folds for vocal hemorrhage, Reinke edema, and hyaluronic acid overinjection: a novel application in the larynx. J Voice. 2018;32(4):492–8. https://doi.org/10.1016/j.jvoice.2017.07.004. Epub 2017 Sep 1. PMID: 28867161.
29. Sataloff RT, Chowdhury F, Portnoy JE, Hawkshaw MJ, Joglekar S. Vocal fold cysts. In: Sataloff RT, Chowdhury F, Portnoy JE, Hawkshaw MJ, Joglekar S, editors. Surgical techniques in otolaryngology—head & neck surgery: laryngeal surgery. London: JP Medical Ltd; 2013. p. 61–71.
30. Hamdan AL, Mourad M, Barazi R, Semaan ZM, Feghali PAR, Ghzayel L. Office-based blue laser therapy for vocal fold cysts: a case series and review of the literature. J Voice. 2025:S0892-1997(25)00097-9. https://doi.org/10.1016/j.jvoice.2025.03.005. PMID: 40148205.
31. Hamdan AL, Sataloff RT, Ramadan O, Eichorn D, Hawkshaw MJ. Blue laser therapy for vocal fold varices and ectasia. In: Hamdan AL, Sataloff RT, Ramadan O, Eichorn D, Hawkshaw MJ, editors. Blue laser surgery in laryngology. Cham: Springer; 2023. p. 15–26.
32. Woo P. Office-based laryngeal procedures. Otolaryngol Clin North Am. 2006;39(1):111–33. https://doi.org/10.1016/j.otc.2005.11.008. PMID: 16469659.
33. Abitbol J, Abitbol P. Surgical management of nonneoplastic vocal fold lesions: laser versus cold knife excision. Curr Opin Otolaryngol Head Neck Surg. 2000;8(6):514–23.
34. Hantzakos A, Dikkers FG, Giovanni A, Benninger MS, Remacle M, Sjögren EV, Woo P. Vocal fold scars: a common classification proposal by the American Laryngological Association and European Laryngological Society. Eur Arch Otorrinolaringol. 2019;276:2289–92.
35. Gale N, Poljak M, Zidar N. Update from the 4th edition of the World Health Organization classification of head and neck tumours: what is new in the 2017 WHO blue book for tumours of the hypopharynx, larynx, trachea and parapharyngeal space. Head Neck Pathol. 2017;11(1):23–32.

36. Cui W, Xu W, Yang Q, Hu R. Clinicopathological parameters associated with histological background and recurrence after surgical intervention of vocal cord leukoplakia. Medicine. 2017;96(22):e7033.
37. Isenberg JS, Crozier DL, Dailey SH. Institutional and comprehensive review of laryngeal leukoplakia. Ann Otol Rhinol Laryngol. 2008;117(1):74–9.
38. Park JC, Altman KW, Prasad VM, Broadhurst M, Akst LM. Laryngeal leukoplakia: state of the art review. Otolaryngol Head Neck Surg. 2021;164(6):1153–9.
39. Chen M, Li C, Yang Y, Cheng L, Wu H. A morphological classification for vocal fold leukoplakia. Braz J Otorhinolaryngol. 2019;85:588–96.
40. Li J, Xu W, Cheng LY. Application of stroboscopy and narrow band imaging endoscopy in the diagnosis of vocal cord leukoplakia. Zhonghua er bi yan hou tou Jing wai ke za zhi = Chin J Otorhinolaryngol Head Neck Surg. 2017;52(11):806–11.
41. El-Demerdash A, Fawaz SA, Sabri SM, Sweed A, Rabie H. Sensitivity and specificity of stroboscopy in preoperative differentiation of dysplasia from early invasive glottic carcinoma. Eur Arch Otorrinolaringol. 2015;272(5):1189–93.
42. Mehlum CS, Rosenberg T, Groentved AM, Dyrvig AK, Godballe C. Can videostroboscopy predict early glottic cancer? A systematic review and meta-analysis. Laryngoscope. 2016;126(9):2079–84.
43. Ni XG, He S, Xu ZG, Gao L, Lu N, Yuan Z, et al. Endoscopic diagnosis of laryngeal cancer and precancerous lesions by narrow band imaging. J Laryngol Otol. 2011;125(3):288–96.
44. Donne AJ, Hampson L, Homer JJ, Hampson IN. The role of HPV type in recurrent respiratory papillomatosis. Int J Pediatr Otorhinolaryngol. 2010;74(1):7–14. https://doi.org/10.1016/j.ijporl.2009.09.004. Epub 2009 Oct 1. PMID: 19800138.
45. Formánek M, Jančatová D, Komínek P, Matoušek P, Zeleník K. Laryngopharyngeal reflux and herpes simplex virus type 2 are possible risk factors for adult-onset recurrent respiratory papillomatosis (prospective case–control study). Clin Otolaryngol. 2017;42(3):597–601.
46. Sataloff RT. Structural abnormalities of the larynx. In: Sataloff RT, editor. Professional voice: the science and art of clinical care, 3-volume set. San Diego (CA): Plural Publishing; 2017. p. 1533–86.
47. Tjon Pian Gi RE, Halmos GB, van Hemel BM, van den Heuvel ER, van der Laan BF, Plaat BE, et al. Narrow band imaging is a new technique in visualization of recurrent respiratory papillomatosis. Laryngoscope. 2012;122(8):1826–30.
48. Williamson AJ, Bondje S. Glottic cancer. InStatPearls [Internet] 2023. StatPearls Publishing.
49. American Cancer Society. Laryngeal and hypopharyngeal cancer risk factors [Internet]. Atlanta (GA): American Cancer Society; [updated 2023 Jul 10; cited 2025 May 15]. https://www.cancer.org/cancer/types/laryngeal-and-hypopharyngeal-cancer/causes-risks-prevention/risk-factors.html.
50. Zeitels SM, Burns JA, Lopez-Guerra G, Anderson RR, Hillman RE. Photoangiolytic laser treatment of early glottic cancer: a new management strategy. Ann Otol Rhinol Laryngol Suppl. 2008;199:3–24. https://doi.org/10.1177/00034894081170s701. PMID: 18710131.
51. Vasudevan SS, Bryan E, Ericksen E, Alla A, Asarkar AA, Olinde L, Katz S, Nathan CA. Transoral laser microsurgery versus radiotherapy for T1–T2 glottic cancer with anterior commissure involvement: a systematic review and meta-analysis. Laryngoscope. 2025;135:1861.
52. Sanabria A, Chaves ALF, Kowalski LP, et al. Organ preservation with chemoradiation in advanced laryngeal cancer: the problem of generalizing results from randomized controlled trials. Auris Nasus Larynx. 2017;44(1):18–25.

Part III

Impact of Vaping on Voice

Prevalence of Voice Disorders in E-Cigarette Users

6

Prevalence of Hoarseness and Voice Characteristics in E-Cigarette Smokers

Voice disorders are common in the general population. The lifetime prevalence varies, with a higher rate being noted among professional voice users and those who rely on their voice to make a living. In a cross-sectional analysis of 14,795 young adults between the ages of 24 and 34 years, Bainbridge et al. noted that 6% had a voice problem that lasted at least 3 days during the past 12 months [1]. In a retrospective analysis of insurance claims that included 536,943 participants, Cohen et al. reported a point prevalence of dysphonia in 0.98% of the cases. The prevalence was higher in females compared to males and in the elderly (above the age of 70 years) compared to youngsters [2]. Benninger et al. investigated the prevalence of voice disorders using the Commercial and Medicare Market Scan databases and noted an increase over the years associated with rising healthcare costs [3].

Many predisposing factors for voice disorders have been identified, one of which is smoking. Numerous investigations indicate that smoking increases the risk of dysphonia. In a systematic review of the risk factors for voice disorders among non-university teachers, Jiang et al. found that smoking was a significant contributing factor, with an odds ratio of 1.31. Other risk factors for voice disorders included respiratory allergies, acid reflux, voice abuse, and noise [4]. Using the national cross-sectional survey of the Korean population, Byeon et al. found that current smokers had an increased risk for voice problems and laryngeal disorders in comparison to non-smokers (odds ratios of 1.77 and 1.56, respectively) [5]. In a cross-sectional study that included 7941 participants, the same authors reported that past smokers and current smokers were more likely to have organic voice disorders compared to non-smokers (odds ratios of 2.97 vs. 3.22, respectively) [6].

The change in voice quality secondary to smoking is often substantiated by alterations in acoustic measures. Awan reported a significant difference in the Dysphonia Severity Index—an objective and quantitative tool based on the combination of

A.-l. Hamdan, *E-Cigarette Smoking, Voice, and Health*, https://doi.org/10.1007/978-3-032-04913-1_6

acoustic and aerodynamic voice measures such as highest frequency (F_0), lowest intensity (I-Low), maximum phonation time (MPT), and jitter—between smokers and non-smokers, mostly due to a decrease in the high fundamental frequency. The authors ascribed the decrease in fundamental frequency and the contracted vocal range to an increase in vocal fold mass due to smoking [7]. Byeon and Cha conducted a meta-analysis on the effect of smoking on subjective and objective voice measures and noted a significant difference in the fundamental frequency and maximum phonation time between smokers and non-smokers. The analysis, which included nine papers, concluded that smoking had a moderate effect on vocal pitch and upper airflow measurements [8]. In another study on the impact of smoking and other confounding factors on voice, Lustosa Pinto et al. reported that smokers had a higher noise-to-harmonic ratio and perturbation parameters than non-smokers, and a higher prevalence of throat-related symptoms such as cough and throat clearing. The authors stressed the etiologic role of confounding factors such as reflux disease in the exacerbation of these symptoms and in altering the acoustic measures. Smokers are also more likely to exhibit abnormal laryngeal findings [9]. Pinar et al. conducted a multidimensional voice assessment on 109 adults and noted the presence of vocal fold erythema with asymmetry and aperiodicity in vocal fold vibration on stroboscopy. Smokers ($n = 59$) had a significantly lower maximum phonation time in comparison to non-smokers ($n = 51$) [10].

In 2006, the e-cigarette was introduced to the United States market with the premise that it is less hazardous to health than conventional cigarettes [11]. Despite advertising it as a safer alternative to conventional smoking, there was a rising concern among healthcare providers about the safety of e-cigarette smoking. With the sharp increase in its use, particularly among adolescents and teenagers, there is a growing number of reports highlighting the adverse effects of e-cigarette smoking on various systems in the body, including the phonatory system. Numerous studies indicate that e-cigarette smokers have an increased risk for voice disorders compared to non-smokers, albeit to a lesser extent than conventional smokers. Lechien et al. reported a 55-year-old woman who presented with persistent aphonia and throat pain that started following the inhalation of hot vapor while using e-cigarettes. Her symptoms evolved to include a feeling of sticky mucus, repetitive throat clearing, and globus sensation. Her Voice Handicap Index at presentation was 60, and auditory perceptual evaluation revealed grade 3 dysphonia, grade 2 roughness, and grade 3 breathiness (G3R2B3). The laryngeal examination showed signs of laryngopharyngeal reflux disease and a left vocal fold lesion/ulceration. A biopsy of the lesion showed a reactive scar with negative antibody markers for mucin, Desmim, Beta-catenin, and other factors. The diagnosis of vapor-induced injury to the vocal folds was suggested, and treatment using proton pump inhibitors and antacids was initiated in addition to dietary behavioral modification. The patient did well in 3–9 months after treatment with resolution of her symptoms [12]. Tuhanioglu et al. conducted a cross-sectional study looking at the voice characteristics of e-cigarette smokers in comparison to conventional cigarette users and non-smokers. Their results showed a higher mean Voice Handicap Index 10 score in conventional cigarette users vs. e-cigarette users and controls. Similarly, the mean shimmer values were higher in the conventional cigarette users group compared to the other two groups (3.81 ± 2.71 for conventional cigarette smokers vs. 2.60 ± 0.95 for e-cigarette users and 2.67 ± 0.83 for non-smokers). The authors concluded that e-cigarettes had a milder impact on voice in comparison to conventional cigarettes [13]. Dealino and Dela Cruz reported no significant difference in the total (Voice Handicap Index) VHI scores between e-cigarette smokers and conventional smokers (8.85 ± 7.64 for the conventional cigarette smokers and 11.12 ± 12.86 for the e-cigarette smokers, p-value = 0.44). Similarly, no significant differences were observed between the two groups across the VHI subscales—functional, physical, and emotional. Using a cut-off of 18 for the VHI, 11.54% of the conventional cigarette smokers had voice impairment vs. 23.08% in the e-cigarette group (p value = 0.17) [14]. Hamdan et al. investigated the impact of heated-cigarette smoking on voice using the Voice-Handicap Index-10 and the Visual Analog Scale in a cohort of 282 subjects who were asked to fill out a survey distributed by email. The results showed that heated cigarette smokers had higher grades of voice changes and fatigue than non-smokers. Moreover, e-cigarette users had a higher mean VHI-10 score in comparison to non-smokers, and a larger number had an abnormal VHI-10 score [15]. Last but not least, Korrami et al. reported a 29-year-old man with a history of daily use of e-cigarettes who presented with hoarseness, sore throat, dysphagia, and dyspnea. Laryngeal examination revealed swelling of the epiglottis and narrowing of the airway. The findings on examination were consistent with the lateral neck soft tissue radiograph showing the thumb sign. The work-up for viral and bacterial infections, namely COVID-19 and streptococcus, was negative. The patient was treated with steroids and antibiotics, following which he recovered completely [16].

Pathophysiology of Voice and Laryngeal Disorders in E-Cigarette Smokers

The pathophysiology of voice disorders in e-cigarette users is complex and multifactorial. Studies have shown that the e-cigarette aerosol can cause direct damage to the vocal fold and laryngeal mucosal lining. Salturk et al. reported vocal fold mucosal hyperplasia and metaplasia following exposure of albino rats to electronic nicotine delivery system vapor for 1 h a day for 4 weeks. Notably, one case of epithelial metaplasia was reported in the control group. Although there was no significant difference in the prevalence of these histologic changes between the study group and controls, the authors highlighted the need for studies on larger cohorts and prolonged vapor exposure to draw valid conclusions regarding the long-term effects of e-cigarette smoking [17]. Lungova et al. investigated the impact of a 1-week e-cigarette vapor extract exposure on human-engineered vocal fold mucosa and noted alteration in mucosal homeostasis and epithelial barrier function. There was thinning of the mucosal lining, epithelial erosion, and damage to luminal cells. The authors also noted alteration in the expression of membrane-associated mucin and increased production of chemokines implicated in the recruitment of eosinophils [18]. Mucin is a protective glycoprotein that also helps in the lubrication of the vocal folds and maintenance of moisture [19]. Another goal of their in vitro study was to examine the mucosal cells' response for 1,3, and 7 days following cessation of exposure to the e-cigarette vapor. The results showed intense epithelial remodeling associated with the expansion of P63, among other elements such as cytokeratin 14. In conclusion, the authors stressed the threat of vaping on vocal fold mucosal health and the need for increased public awareness [20].

The impact of e-cigarette smoke is not limited to the vocal fold mucosal lining. It also affects the submucosal constituents of the lamina propria. Martinez et al. evaluated the impact of e-cigarette vapor with or without nicotine on cultured human vocal fold fibroblasts and noted a reduction in the viability of these cells, albeit to a lesser extent than that of cigarette smoke extract. There was no DNA damage or changes in gene expression. The authors concluded that e-cigarette vapor extract is less harmful than cigarette smoke extract and that further studies are needed to understand the vocal folds' response to e-cigarette aerosol [20]. In 2024, Grossman et al. investigated the effect of a specific brand of e-cigarettes on the extracellular matrix of the vocal folds and its constituents and showed a decrease in the inflammatory marker gene expression, namely cyclooxygenase and Interleukin, during static and dynamic conditions. On the other hand, there were no changes in HA production, fibrogenic markers, or angiogenic factors except for downregulation in VEGF-D gene expression during vibration [21].

E-cigarette smoke may also impact the voice by affecting other systems in the body aside from the vocal folds, including the various components of the phonatory apparatus. E-cigarettes may impair breathing, which is the power source of voice production. Numerous reports indicate that e-cigarette users are more likely to complain of respiratory symptoms such as cough, dyspnea, and wheeze than non-smokers [22, 23]. The work-up of these patients often reveals alteration in pulmonary function testing in rare cases, and abnormalities on radiologic imaging of the chest in severe cases [24, 25]. Investigators have also shown that vaping can exacerbate pre-existing lower airway diseases such as asthma and chronic obstructive airway disease and increases the risk of developing these conditions [26]. More details on the impact of e-cigarette on the respiratory system and the pathophysiology of breathing disorders in e-cigarette users are discussed in Chap. 7. Vaping can also affect the sinonasal tract and oral cavity, which act as resonators for the vocal signal. Numerous studies showed that vaping increases the risk for allergic rhinitis and chronic rhinosinusitis. E-cigarette users are more likely to suffer from sinonasal symptoms such as nasal congestion, post-nasal drip, and headache [27]. These symptoms are mostly ascribed to alterations in the ciliary beating of the mucosal lining, among other factors. More details on the impact of e-cigarette aerosol on the sinonasal mucosa are available in Chap. 9. The impact of vaping on the oral cavity, which is a main resonant cavity, is also substantial. The oral cavity is the first anatomic area exposed to e-cigarette aerosol. Studies have shown that vaping leads to changes in the oral microbiome, alterations in the composition, and function of saliva. Vaping has also been associated with mucosal lesions and an increase in periodontogenic diseases [28]. More details on the impact of vaping on the oral cavity are present in Chap. 8. E-cigarettes may also affect voice indirectly by exacerbating common risk factors for voice disorders, such as gastro-esophageal and laryngopharyngeal reflux diseases. A review on the link between gastrointestinal disorders and e-cigarette use is available in Chap. 10.

References

1. Bainbridge KE, Roy N, Losonczy KG, Hoffman HJ, Cohen SM. Voice disorders and associated risk markers among young adults in the United States. Laryngoscope. 2017;127(9):2093–9.
2. Cohen SM, Kim J, Roy N, Asche C, Courey M. Prevalence and causes of dysphonia in a large treatment-seeking population. Laryngoscope. 2012;122(2):343–8.
3. Benninger MS, Holy CE, Bryson PC, Milstein CF. Prevalence and occupation of patients presenting with dysphonia in the United States. J Voice. 2017;31(5):594–600.
4. Jiang G, Xu X, Yu K, Tang G, Yang R, Li X. The risk factors of voice disorders in non-university teachers: a systematic review and meta-analysis. J Voice. 2024:S0892-1997(24)00372-2.
5. Byeon H. The association between lifetime cigarette smoking and dysphonia in the Korean general population: findings from a national survey. PeerJ. 2015;3:e912.
6. Byeon H. Relationships among smoking, organic, and functional voice disorders in Korean general population. J Voice. 2015;29(3):312–6.
7. Awan SN. The effect of smoking on the dysphonia severity index in females. Folia Phoniatr Logop. 2011;63(2):65–71.
8. Byeon H, Cha S. Evaluating the effects of smoking on the voice and subjective voice problems using a meta-analysis approach. Sci Rep. 2020;10(1):4720.
9. Pinto AG, Crespo AN, Mourão LF. Influence of smoking isolated and associated to multifactorial aspects in vocal acoustic parameters. Braz J Otorhinolaryngol. 2014;80:60–7.
10. Pinar D, Cincik H, Erkul E, Gungor A. Investigating the effects of smoking on young adult male voice by using multidimensional methods. J Voice. 2016;30(6):721–5.
11. Debbaneh P, Dhir S, Anderson M, Rivero A. Electronic cigarettes: a narrative review and cohort study of electronic cigarette users in the otolaryngology clinic. Perm J. 2022;26(4):85.
12. Lechien JR, Papon JF, Pouliquen C, Hans S. E-cigarette vaping-related vocal fold injury: a case report. J Voice. 2024;38(1):195–6.
13. Tuhanioğlu B, Erkan SO, Özdaş T, Derici Ç, Tüzün K, Şenkal ÖA. The effect of electronic cigarettes on voice quality. J Voice. 2019;33(5):811–e13.
14. Dealino MA, Cruz AP. Dysphonia in smokers of combustible cigarettes and e-cigarettes measured using the Filipino Voice Handicap Index. Philippine J Otolaryngol Head Neck Surg. 2022;37(1):27.
15. Hamdan AL, Daou CA, Yammine Y, Jabbour C, Carapiperis I, Helou V, Ghadieh J, Lechien JR. The effect of heated-cigarette smoking on voice in comparison to combustion-cigarette smoking: self-perceived evaluation. J Laryngol Otol. 2025;139(2):129–33.
16. Khorrami A, Khorrami MA, Gheriani H. Vaping-induced acute epiglottitis: a case report. Int J Emerg Med. 2023;16(1):56.
17. Salturk Z, Çakır Ç, Sünnetçi G, Atar Y, Kumral TL, Yıldırım G, Berkiten G, Uyar Y. Effects of electronic nicotine delivery system on larynx: experimental study. J Voice. 2015;29(5):560–3.
18. Lungova V, Wendt K, Thibeault SL. Exposure to e-cigarette vapor extract induces vocal fold epithelial injury and triggers intense mucosal remodeling. Dis Model Mech. 2022;15(8):dmm049476.
19. Peters G, Wendler O, Böhringer D, Gostian AO, Müller SK, Canziani H, Hesse N, Semmler M, Berry DA, Kniesburges S, Peukert W. Human laryngeal mucus from the vocal folds: rheological characterization by particle tracking microrheology and oscillatory shear rheology. Appl Sci. 2021;11(7):3011.

20. Martinez JD, Easwaran M, Ramirez D, Erickson-DiRenzo E. Effects of electronic (e)-cigarette vapor and cigarette smoke in cultured vocal fold fibroblasts. Laryngoscope. 2023;133(1):139–46.
21. Grossmann T, Kirsch A, Gerstenberger C, Steffan B, Gugatschka M. Describing the cellular impact of IQOS™ smoke extract and vibration on human vocal fold fibroblasts. J Voice. 2024;S0892-1997(24):00135-8.
22. Hedman L, Backman H, Stridsman C, Bosson JA, Lundbäck M, Lindberg A, Rönmark E, Ekerljung L. Association of electronic cigarette use with smoking habits, demographic factors, and respiratory symptoms. JAMA Netw Open. 2018;1(3):e180789.
23. Soule EK, Bode KM, Desrosiers AC, Guy M, Breland A, Fagan P. User-perceived negative respiratory symptoms associated with electronic cigarette use. Nicotine Tob Res. 2020;22(Suppl 1):S45–53.
24. Sreedharan S, Mian M, Robertson RA, Rhodes A. Radiological findings of e-cigarette or vaping product use associated lung injury: a systematic review. Heart Lung. 2021;50(5):736–41.
25. Honeycutt L, Huerne K, Miller A, Wennberg E, Filion KB, Grad R, Gershon AS, Ells C, Gore G, Benedetti A, Thombs B. A systematic review of the effects of e-cigarette use on lung function. NPJ Prim Care Respir Med. 2022;32(1):45.
26. Yang X, Che W, Zhang L, Zhang H, Chen X. Chronic airway inflammatory diseases and e-cigarette use: a review of health risks and mechanisms. Eur J Med Res. 2025;30(1):1–2.
27. Rha MS, Cho HJ, Yoon JH, Kim CH. Association between the use of electronic cigarettes and the prevalence of chronic rhinosinusitis and allergic rhinitis: a nationwide cross-sectional study. Rhinology. 2022;60(1):20–8.
28. Charde P, Ali K, Hamdan N. Effects of e-cigarette smoking on periodontal health: a scoping review. PLOS Glob Public Health. 2024;4(3):e0002311.

7 Breathing Disorders in E-Cigarette Users and Their Impact on Voice

Respiratory Symptoms in E-Cigarette Users

E-cigarettes produce an aerosol that contains several ingredients, including nicotine, propylene glycol, and glycerol. Other detected compounds include acetone, toluene, acetaldehyde, formaldehyde, and metallic nanoparticles [1]. These constituents may have adverse effects on health and various systems in the body, including the respiratory system.

Prevalence of Respiratory Symptoms in Vapers

There is ubiquity of reports in the literature suggesting that the use of e-cigarettes leads to an array of respiratory symptoms. In a study that included 30,272 participants, Hedman et al. reported a higher prevalence of respiratory symptoms among dual smokers who used traditional and e-cigarettes in comparison to non-smokers, former smokers, and e-cigarette users alone. The most commonly reported symptoms were chronic cough, wheezing, and sputum production [2]. Soule et al. identified eight clusters of self-perceived symptoms associated with the use of e-cigarettes, which included respiratory symptoms. The most common were dyspnea and cough. Other systemic complaints included body fatigue, throat dryness, xerostomia, excessive phlegm, and dysgeusia [3]. Baweja et al. surveyed the views of experienced e-cigarette users and noted respiratory symptoms among the negative effects associated with vaping. A commonly used term in their survey was "exacerbation of asthma symptoms," in addition to many other systemic complaints such as headache and increased heart rate [4]. These reports concur with a study by Khosravi et al. that showed transient bronchial constriction more than 2 min following exposure to a single puff of e-cigarette aerosol [5].

In line with the above, numerous authors also showed that e-cigarette use exacerbates pre-existing lung diseases. Using a telephone survey that included 8087

A.-l. Hamdan, *E-Cigarette Smoking, Voice, and Health*,
https://doi.org/10.1007/978-3-032-04913-1_7

participants, Willis et al. noted a significant association between e-cigarette smoking and chronic pulmonary disorders with an adjusted odds ratio of 2.58 [6]. In a review on the impact of e-cigarettes on respiratory function, Thirion-Romero et al. reported excess mucus and airway irritation as common complaints. The authors also noted that vapor smoking exacerbated the respiratory symptoms of asthma, chronic obstructive airway disease, and cystic fibrosis [7]. McConnell investigated the link between e-cigarette smoking and chronic bronchitis in 502 e-cigarette smokers and noted a 2.02-fold increase in risk of bronchitis in current users in comparison to never-users. The risk of bronchitis also increased by 1.85-fold among past-users in comparison to never-users. The authors highlighted the higher prevalence of bronchitis symptoms in past and current smokers, even after adjusting for confounders [8]. Cho and Paik investigated the link between e-cigarette smoking and asthma in a cohort of 35,904 high school students. Using a self-reported questionnaire, the authors noted a higher prevalence of asthma in current e-cigarette users in comparison to former e-cigarette users and non-smokers (3.9% vs. 2.2% vs. 1.7%, respectively) and a higher adjusted odds ratio (adjusted OR = 2.74). The study concluded that e-cigarette smoking may increase the risk of asthma [9]. Schweitzer et al. examined the association between asthma and e-cigarette smoking using a survey that included 6089 students in 33 schools. The results showed that current e-cigarette users were at a higher risk of having current asthma (adjusted odds ratio of 1.48) and previously having asthma (adjusted odds ratio of 1.22). The authors concluded that there was an independent association between e-cigarette use and asthma, with a higher prevalence noted in Blacks, Native Hawaiians, Filipinos, and Pacific islanders in comparison to Caucasian and Asian Americans [10]. Reid et al. examined the rate of e-cigarette smoking among middle and high school students and noted that the current use of tobacco was higher in asthmatic students in comparison to those without asthma, and that e-cigarette was the most common tobacco type used in middle and high school students with a prevalence of 7.9% and 19.6%, respectively [11].

The respiratory symptoms of e-cigarette users are often associated with abnormal pulmonary function tests (PFT). Vardavas et al. showed a significant decrease in the fraction of exhaled nitric oxide (Feno) and a significant increase in respiratory impedance and respiratory resistance at 5, 10, and 20 Hz following e-cigarette use for 5 min [12]. In an animal study, Larcombe et al. reported a decrease in lung function (parenchymal) at high trans-respiratory pressure and at functional residual capacity following the exposure of BALB/C mice to e-cigarette aerosol for 8 weeks. Moreover, when glycerin-based e-cigarette aerosol was used, the airway exhibited a hyper-response to methacholine challenge [13]. Meo et al. investigated the effect of e-cigarettes on lung function in 30 males. The results showed a decrease in forced expiratory flow and forced expiratory ratio (FEV1/FVC) in the e-cigarette group compared to a healthy control group matched by age, socioeconomic factors, height, and weight. Given that the abstinence time from smoking was at least 1 h before testing, the impairment in lung function was suggestive of an obstructive peripheral airway disease [14]. On the other hand, it is worth noting that the effect of e-cigarette use on pulmonary function seems to be less severe than that of traditional smoking.

Flouris et al. assessed the impact of e-cigarette smoking on pulmonary function in 15 smokers following a session of active smoking of tobacco cigarettes and a session of active smoking of e-cigarettes. Although both types of smoking had a similar effect on serum cotinine, e-cigarette use was found to have a minimal and non-significant impact on lung function (% FEV1/FVC reduction) compared to tobacco smoking. Passive e-cigarette smoking in a control group also did not impact PFT significantly [15]. Ferrari et al. assessed the impact of nicotine-free e-cigarette (specific brand) on the lungs of smokers and noted a significant effect on FEV1 and FEF25 [16]. In a crossover and placebo-controlled trial, Boulay et al. investigated the effect of 1 h vaping nicotine-free and flavor-free e-liquid on breathing. The results showed a non-significant impact on respiratory mechanics and lung function of healthy or asthmatic participants. It is important to note that the vaping session was conducted in a controlled environment using a contaminant-free and high-grade mixture of propylene glycol and glycerol [17].

Pathophysiology of Respiratory Symptoms in E-Cigarette Users

The pathophysiology of respiratory symptoms and signs in e-cigarette smokers is complex. Several suggested mechanisms have been proposed, the most commonly cited being alterations in the immune system, inflammation, and an increase in oxidative stress. A culmination of these factors is probably the cause of breathing problems in e-cigarette users.

Impact of E-Cigarette Use on the Immune System

The premise that e-cigarette use has an adverse effect on the immune system stems from numerous reports showing an increased rate of respiratory infection in e-cigarette users and high resistance to conventional treatment in affected patients. This is not surprising, knowing that the respiratory tract epithelium plays a role in the defense mechanism against inhaled toxins. E-cigarette use has been shown to decrease epithelial mucociliary function and increase microbial activity and bacterial growth. Carson et al. investigated the structure and function of nasal epithelium following exposure to e-cigarette smoke and noted a decrease in ciliary beating frequency that was associated with a mild elevation in nitrous oxide. The decline in ciliary beating recovered within an hour after cessation of the exposure. The authors alluded that chronic exposure to e-cigarette vapor may predispose to chronic pathology secondary to these epithelial changes [18]. Ghosh et al. investigated the epithelial cell barrier following sub-chronic exposure to e-cigarette smoke, including other forms of smoke, using human bronchial epithelial cells in an air–liquid interface. They found a decrease in trans-electrical epithelial resistance by 60%, and a decrease in cilia beating frequency by 59% following exposure to e-cigarette smoke (1.2% concentration of nicotine). The authors concluded that sub-chronic exposure to e-cigarette aerosol disrupts the epithelial barrier and can be toxic [19]. The adverse effects of e-cigarette aerosol on ciliary function and epithelial barrier are surmounted by its impact on certain pathogens, increasing their capacity to proliferate and invade tissue. Sussan et al. investigated the effect of e-cigarettes on the pulmonary defense mechanism in a mouse model and noted a significant impairment in bacterial clearance following exposure to *Streptococcus pneumonia*. They also found a surge in lung viral titers and an increased mortality following exposure to influenza A virus [20]. Miyashita et al. reported an increase in platelet-activating factor receptor (PAFR) expression in the nasal epithelium of adults exposed to e-cigarette vapor for 5 min. In an animal model using mice, the authors also showed an increase in PAFR expression and colonization of pneumococci in the nasopharynx. The increased colonization was ascribed to the fact that pneumococci co-opt PAFR to better adhere to airway cells. The study concluded that e-cigarette vapor exposure increases the risk of pneumococcal infection [21].

E-cigarette use has also been shown to suppress immune cell function. The alveolar macrophages (AM), which are innate immune cells of the lower airway responsible for clearing pathogens and debris, are also affected. Numerous studies showed that their capacity to phagocytose bacteria and foreign particles is impaired. Hwang et al. investigated the effect of e-cigarette vapor on human epithelial cells and found a decrease in the antimicrobial activity of alveolar macrophages and other immune cells toward *Staphylococcus aureus*. Inhalation of e-vapor led to an increase in *Staphylococcus aureus* colonization, thus exacerbating the virulence of the colonizing bacteria [22]. Ween et al. explored the effect of e-cigarettes on the function of macrophages in human airway epithelial cells of healthy non-smokers and noted that e-liquid flavoring, nicotine, and their combination significantly reduced phagocytosis of non-typical hemophiles (NTHi) bacteria, similar to cigarette smoke extract (CSE) [23]. Scott et al. investigated the effect of e-cigarette liquid (ECL) and e-cigarette vapor condensate (ECVC) on alveolar macrophages using alveolar macrophages isolated from human lung tissue and THP-1 human macrophages and noted a decrease in cell viability. ECVC was found to be more toxic than ECL and can lead to an increase in cell necrosis and apoptosis. The addition of nicotine to e-cigarette vapor worsened AM function. When exposed to a sub-lethal concentration of ECVC, AM also exhibited a decrease in capacity to phagocytose [24]. Madison et al. reported aberrant phospholipids in AM of mice exposed to electronic nicotine delivery system vapor for 4 months. The authors also noted downregulation of the immune function of macrophages in their defense following exposure to viral pathogens [25].

Studies also indicate that e-cigarette use affects the activity of neutrophils, which play an important role in the defense mechanism against infection. Inhalation of e-cigarette aerosol has been shown to impair neutrophil function and increase Neutrophil Extracellular Trap (NET) formation [26]. NETosis is a defense mechanism whereby neutrophils release DNA after lysis into the extracellular environment with the purpose of immobilizing bacteria [27, 28]. Using sputum samples, Reidels et al. reported an increase in NET-related proteins in e-cigarette users. Although NETs are useful in clearing pathogens, their rise can be damaging to the pulmonary epithelium [28]. In a review on the emerging role of NET, Twaddell et al. noted that NETs can be cytotoxic to lung endothelium and epithelium [29]. In patients with chronic lung diseases such as COPD and cystic fibrosis, an abundance of NET has been identified and is considered an index of lung injury.

E-Cigarette-Induced Inflammation and Oxidative Stress

Numerous investigators showed an association between E-cigarette use, inflammatory markers, and markers of oxidative stress [30, 31]. In 2014, Lim and Kim examined the effect of intratracheal e-cigarette solution injections in mice and found an increase in the infiltration of inflammatory cells into the airway, which worsened the asthmatic airway inflammation and airway hyperresponsiveness [32]. In 2015, Lerner et al. noted that exposure of airway epithelial cells to electronic nicotine delivery systems (ENDS) led to an increase in inflammatory markers such as cytokines and IL-6 and IL-8, and that exposure of human lung fibroblasts to ENDS/E-liquids resulted in morphologic changes and increased susceptibility to loss of cell viability. Exposure of mice to aerosols also resulted in an increase in inflammatory cytokines and a decrease in lung glutathione levels. The authors concluded that e-cigarette vapor and juice increased oxidative stress and inflammation, which may increase the risk for health disorders [33]. In 2016, Husari et al. investigated the impact of e-cigarette smoke on the lungs in an animal model. Mice were exposed to e-cigarette aerosol for 6 h per day for 3 days, and lung injury was measured using various parameters, including expression of inflammatory markers, oxidative stress, and cell death. The authors noted only an increase in IL-1b. In contrast to mice who were exposed to cigarette smoke, e-cigarette aerosol exposure did not lead to albumin leak, oxidative stress, and cell death [34]. In 2018, Scotts et al. conducted a study where AM were treated with ECVC with and without nicotine and found an increase in pro-inflammatory markers, namely tumor necrosis factor alpha, interleukin-6, and matrix metalloproteinase 9. The adverse effect was almost reversed when treated with the antioxidant N-acetyl-cysteine [24]. In 2018, Reidel et al. investigated the effects of e-cigarettes on the airway using sputum samples and noted an increase in the concentration of mucins MUCSAC. Results also showed an increase in oxidative stress-related proteins and levels of innate defense proteins. The authors concluded that there was an alteration in the airway secretions' innate defense proteins [28]. In 2020, in a cross-sectional study that included 73 participants, Song et al. reported higher levels of inflammatory biomarkers in bronchoalveolar lavage and brushings of e-cigarette smokers compared to non-smokers. On the other hand, these levels were lower in comparison to cigarette smokers, suggesting a less toxic effect [35]. On the other hand, Song et al. found that the differential gene expression of bronchial epithelial cells in e-cigarette smokers was almost similar to never-smokers [35].

These reports are not surprising, knowing that e-cigarette use has been linked to chronic inflammatory airway diseases and given the presence of free radicals in e-cigarette aerosols.

Using electron paramagnetic resonance spectroscopy, Goel et al. examined EC aerosols and found highly oxidizing free radicals. The authors highlighted the toxic risk of these short-lived free radicals on health [36]. Haddad et al. measured ROS emission in sub-ohm and supra-ohm electronic cigarettes and noted a variation in relation to power per unit area, heating design, and composition of the liquid that is heated in terms of propylene glycol to vegetable glycerin. An increase in VG concentration results in an increase in ROS [37].

E-Cigarette-Induced Lung Injury

Acute respiratory illness related to vaping was recognized in 2019 by numerous local and state health departments in the United States. Both the Food and Drug administration and the US Centers for Disease Control and Prevention coined the term "E-cigarette or vaping product use-associated lung injury" (EVALI) to describe a systemic illness associated with bilateral lung infiltrates in patients with recent history of vaping within the last 3 months and in the absence of other causes such as infections autoimmune diseases or malignancies [38, 39]. EVALI is more common in men with a mean age of 23 years and has a worse prognosis in older patients [40]. Patients present mostly with respiratory symptoms such as cough and shortness of breath and constitutional symptoms such as body fatigue and fever, with evidence of pulmonary infiltrates on chest imaging [41]. Other presenting complaints include gastrointestinal symptoms such as diarrhea and abdominal pain [41–44]. Based on a report by Layden et al., which included 98 cases, respiratory and constitutional symptoms were common in 97% and 100% of the cases, respectively [42, 45]. On physical examination, the patient may show signs of hypoxemia in addition to tachypnea, tachycardia, and a possible decrease in breath sounds on chest auscultation [42]. Laboratory tests can show leukocytosis and an increase in inflammatory biomarkers such as CRP.

Although the majority of patients with EVALI recover using supportive measures, many may need mechanical ventilation and often endure major complications leading to death. In the study by Layden et al., 265 of the affected patients were intubated. Based on the US Centers for Disease Control, 54 deaths have been reported in 2019, with a median age of 53 [39]. The majority of cases reported using products containing nicotine or THC, suggesting a link between these ingredients and exacerbation of disease [40]. Other incriminating ingredients included vitamin E-acetate. Blount et al. conducted isotope dilution mass spectrometry on bronchoalveolar-lavage fluids of 51 patients diagnosed with or suspected of having EVALI. The analysis revealed vitamin E-acetate in 94% of the cases in addition to other ingredients such as THC or its metabolites [46]. Vitamin E acetate can decompose at high temperature (boiling point 220 °C) to ketene, which is highly toxic and damaging to ling tissue [47].

Several patterns of lung injury have been suggested, with the most common being organizing pneumonia (OP) and diffuse alveolar damage (DAD). Imaging patterns associated with OP range from nodule formation to diffuse hazy opacities, often referred to as a ground glass appearance. This latter can be bilateral and involves the upper, middle, and lower lung parenchyma. Areas of lobular sparing may be seen centrally, peripherally, and along the peri-broncho-vascular interstitium. Another common radiologic sign is centrilobular nodules, which are often attributed to a hypersensitivity reaction and or pulmonary hemorrhage. Imaging patterns suggestive of DAD include also ground glass opacity and septal thickening with consolidation of the lower lobe. These signs are mostly seen during the exudative phase of the disease during which patients are very ill and may be in need for ventilatory assistance. With the progression of the disease to the organizing phase, other signs may prevail such as reticulation and volume loss. A less common form of pneumonia that has also been associated with EVALI is acute eosinophilic pneumonia. Acute eosinophilic pneumonia is characterized by acute lung injury secondary to eosinophilic degranulation, which leads to an increase in vascular permeability and edema. Although the computerized tomography (CT) findings can be similar to those seen in DAD and OP, acute eosinophilic pneumonia is suspected in the presence of pleural effusion suggestive of fluid overload. The high concentration of eosinophils (more than 25%) in the bronchoalveolar lavage in the absence of infection or febrile illness, and adequate response to steroid are also suggestive of this disease [48, 49]. Patients with EVALI may also exhibit symptoms and signs of pulmonary hemorrhage. Findings on CT include nodules, consolidation, and ground-glass opacity. Other radiologic signs include tree-in-bud configuration and thickening of septa [50]. Cyto-histopathologic examination of bronchoalveolar lavage fluid invariably show evidence of inflammatory cells and lipid-laden macrophages, a finding commonly associated with endogenous lipid pneumonia [51]. Saqi et al. conducted a cytologic evaluation of broncho-alveolar lavage specimens from EVALI patients and noted that macrophages had distended cytoplasm and fine cytoplasmic vacuoles. These cytoplasmic vacuoles could represent cellular lipid material derived from injured epithelial cells [52].

Despite all the above, it is important to note that EVALI is a diagnosis of exclusion. Ruling out an infectious process using a respiratory syncytial panel, blood and sputum cultures is an essential diagnostic criteria bases on CDC [41]. Inability to rule out an infection or a suspicion that of a superimposed infection makes the diagnosis probable but not certain. Butt et al. examined the lung biopsies of 17 patients suspected of having EVALI, 11 of whom diagnosed with EVALI, and noted common histopathologic patterns in all cases such as OP, DAD, and acute fibrinous pneumonitis. Other histologic findings included pneumocyte vacuolization and the presence of foamy macrophages. There was also prominence of neutrophils [53]. Mukhopadhyay et al. reported the lung biopsy findings of 8 patients diagnosed with EVALI based on radiologic evidence of bilateral ground glass opacities and a negative workup of other etiologies. Similar to the findings of Butt et al., there was evidence of DAD and OP with histopathologic features of fibrinous exudates, hyaline membranes, and interstitial organization among other findings, all suggestive of an acute lung injury pattern [54].

Impact of E-Cigarette-Induced Respiratory Dysfunction on Voice

There are no studies on the impact of e-cigarette-induced respiratory dysfunction on voice, but there is ubiquity of reports on the paramount role of breathing in phonation and the adverse effects of lower airway diseases on voice. Breathing is the power source of phonation and plays a paramount role in vocal fold vibration. Both inspiratory and expiratory muscles contribute to phonation. The diaphragm, in addition to being the most important inspiratory muscle, helps in stabilizing the vocal tract and in adjusting the subglottic pressure during voice production [55–57]. Similarly, movement of the chest wall during expiration is crucial in phonation. Contraction of the internal intercostal muscles assists in regulating airflow across the glottis. A dysfunction in the internal intercostal muscles may hinder the expiratory breathing forces, whereas dysfunction of the external intercostals can affect lung expansion. Limitations in chest wall movement secondary to pain or restrictive pulmonary diseases can impair the ability of the speaker to project his or her voice [58–60].

E-cigarette use has been associated with asthma, which in turn is linked to voice disorders. In a population-based study, which included 19,330 participants, Park et al. reported a higher prevalence of dysphonia and organic laryngeal lesions in asthmatic patients compared to non-asthmatic [61]. In a study on 40 asthmatic patients, Dogan et al. noted that 40% of their study group had an abnormal VHI score. The high self-reported scores were associated with an increase in the acoustic perturbation parameters, jitter and shimmer in women, and an increase in shimmer in men [62]. Hamdan et al. investigated the phonatory symptoms of 31 asthmatic patients and noted a higher prevalence of voice disorders and worse auditory perceptual ratings compared to a control group [63]. Lavy et al. reported cycle-to-cycle irregularities and a decrease in maximum phonation time in 40% and almost 2/3 of their study group, which consisted of 22 asthmatic patients [64]. These findings are often associated with abnormalities on laryngeal examination. Stanton et al. reported functional or structural laryngeal abnormalities in 26 out of 43 asthmatic patients [65]. Dogan et al. reported vocal fold bowing in 25% of the cases and abnormal glottic closure in 25% and 60% of the cases, respectively. Other common stroboscopic findings included irregularities in vocal fold vibration and phase asymmetry in 67.5% and 30% of the cases, respectively [62]. The voice disorders in asthmatic patients can be attributed to many factors, such as impaired breathing and the use of inhaled corticosteroids. Asthmatic patients are known to have an increase in airway resistance and episodic airway obstruction, often associated with a decrease in expiratory peak flow and maximum phonation time. These aerodynamic alterations undoubtedly impact breathing support and control, leading to an increased risk of voice disorders. Similarly, the use of inhaled corticosteroids is a potential cause for dysphonia in asthmatic patients [66]. Using a questionnaire, Ihre et al. reported a positive correlation between vocal symptoms and the use of inhaled cortisone. The most common symptoms were hoarseness, lump sensation, and throat clearing [67].

Many mechanisms have been suggested, including vocal fold muscle-induced atrophy, fungal infection, and mucosal irritation [68].

Chronic obstructive lung disease (COPD) has also been associated with voice and swallowing disorders. Bassi et al. reported COPD as the most common comorbidity in patients with oropharyngeal dysphagia, and Ryu et al. noted an independent association between COPD and dysphonia [69, 70]. The pathophysiology of dysphonia in COPD patients has been based primarily on the use of corticosteroids, which often resulted in "increase of hypotonus" as described by Kozak et al. in their report on the effect of chronic use of inhaled steroids in patients with COPD [71].

References

1. Dinakar C, O'Connor GT. The health effects of electronic cigarettes. N Engl J Med. 2016;375(14):1372–81. https://doi.org/10.1056/NEJMra1502466. PMID: 27705269.
2. Hedman L, Backman H, Stridsman C, Bosson JA, Lundbäck M, Lindberg A, Rönmark E, Ekerljung L. Association of electronic cigarette use with smoking habits, demographic factors, and respiratory symptoms. JAMA Netw Open. 2018;1(3):e180789.
3. Soule EK, Bode KM, Desrosiers AC, Guy M, Breland A, Fagan P. User-perceived negative respiratory symptoms associated with electronic cigarette use. Nicotine Tob Res. 2020;22(Suppl 1):S45–53.
4. Baweja R, Curci KM, Yingst J, Veldheer S, Hrabovsky S, Wilson SJ, Nichols TT, Eissenberg T, Foulds J. Views of experienced electronic cigarette users. Addict Res Theory. 2016;24(1):80–8.
5. Khosravi M, Lin RL, Lee LY. Inhalation of electronic cigarette aerosol induces reflex bronchoconstriction by activation of vagal bronchopulmonary C-fibers. Am J Physiol Lung Cell Mol Physiol. 2018;315(4):L467–75.
6. Wills TA, Pagano I, Williams RJ, Tam EK. E-cigarette use and respiratory disorder in an adult sample. Drug Alcohol Depend. 2019;194:363–70. https://doi.org/10.1016/j.drugalcdep.2018.10.004.
7. Thirión-Romero I, Pérez-Padilla R, Zabert G, Barrientos-Gutiérrez I. Respiratory impact of electronic cigarettes and "low-risk" tobacco. Rev Investig Clin. 2019;71(1):17–27.
8. McConnell R, Barrington-Trimis JL, Wang K, Urman R, Hong H, Unger J, Samet J, Leventhal A, Berhane K. Electronic cigarette use and respiratory symptoms in adolescents. Am J Respir Crit Care Med. 2017;195(8):1043–9.
9. Cho JH, Paik SY. Association between electronic cigarette use and asthma among high school students in South Korea. PLoS One. 2016;11(3):e0151022.
10. Schweitzer RJ, Wills TA, Tam E, Pagano I, Choi K. E-cigarette use and asthma in a multiethnic sample of adolescents. Prev Med. 2017;105:226–31.
11. Reid KM, Forrest JR, Porter L. Tobacco product use among youths with and without lifetime asthma—Florida, 2016. MMWR Morb Mortal Wkly Rep. 2018;67(21):599–601.
12. Vardavas CI, Anagnostopoulos N, Kougias M, Evangelopoulou V, Connolly GN, Behrakis PK. Short-term pulmonary effects of using an electronic cigarette: impact on respiratory flow resistance, impedance, and exhaled nitric oxide. Chest. 2012;141(6):1400–6.
13. Larcombe AN, Janka MA, Mullins BJ, Berry LJ, Bredin A, Franklin PJ. The effects of electronic cigarette aerosol exposure on inflammation and lung function in mice. Am J Physiol Lung Cell Mol Physiol. 2017;313(1):L67–79.
14. Meo SA, Ansary MA, Barayan FR, Almusallam AS, Almehaid AM, Alarifi NS, Alsohaibani TA, Zia I. Electronic cigarettes: impact on lung function and fractional exhaled nitric oxide among healthy adults. Am J Mens Health. 2019;13(1):1557988318806073.

15. Flouris AD, Chorti MS, Poulianiti KP, Jamurtas AZ, Kostikas K, Tzatzarakis MN, Wallace Hayes A, Tsatsakis AM, Koutedakis Y. Acute impact of active and passive electronic cigarette smoking on serum cotinine and lung function. Inhal Toxicol. 2013;25(2):91–101.
16. Ferrari M, Zanasi A, Nardi E, Morselli Labate AM, Ceriana P, Balestrino A, Pisani L, Corcione N, Nava S. Short-term effects of a nicotine-free e-cigarette compared to a traditional cigarette in smokers and non-smokers. BMC Pulm Med. 2015;15:120.
17. Boulay MÈ, Henry C, Bossé Y, Boulet LP, Morissette MC. Acute effects of nicotine-free and flavour-free electronic cigarette use on lung functions in healthy and asthmatic individuals. Respir Res. 2017;18(1):33.
18. Carson JL, Zhou L, Brighton L, Mills KH, Zhou H, Jaspers I, Hazucha M. Temporal structure/function variation in cultured differentiated human nasal epithelium associated with acute single exposure to tobacco smoke or E-cigarette vapor. Inhal Toxicol. 2017;29(3):137–44.
19. Ghosh B, Reyes-Caballero H, Akgün-Ölmez SG, Nishida K, Chandrala L, Smirnova L, Biswal S, Sidhaye VK. Effect of sub-chronic exposure to cigarette smoke, electronic cigarette and waterpipe on human lung epithelial barrier function. BMC Pulm Med. 2020;20(1):216.
20. Sussan TE, Gajghate S, Thimmulappa RK, Ma J, Kim JH, Sudini K, Consolini N, Cormier SA, Lomnicki S, Hasan F, Pekosz A, Biswal S. Exposure to electronic cigarettes impairs pulmonary anti-bacterial and anti-viral defenses in a mouse model. PLoS One. 2015;10(2):e0116861.
21. Miyashita L, Suri R, Dearing E, Mudway I, Dove RE, Neill DR, Van Zyl-Smit R, Kadioglu A, Grigg J. E-cigarette vapour enhances pneumococcal adherence to airway epithelial cells. Eur Respir J. 2018;51(2):1701592.
22. Hwang JH, Lyes M, Sladewski K, Enany S, McEachern E, Mathew DP, Das S, Moshensky A, Bapat S, Pride DT, Ongkeko WM, Crotty Alexander LE. Electronic cigarette inhalation alters innate immunity and airway cytokines while increasing the virulence of colonizing bacteria. J Mol Med (Berl). 2016;94(6):667–79.
23. Ween MP, Whittall JJ, Hamon R, Reynolds PN, Hodge SJ. Phagocytosis and inflammation: exploring the effects of the components of E-cigarette vapor on macrophages. Physiol Rep. 2017;5(16):e13370.
24. Scott A, Lugg ST, Aldridge K, Lewis KE, Bowden A, Mahida RY, Grudzinska FS, Dosanjh D, Parekh D, Foronjy R, Sapey E, Naidu B, Thickett DR. Pro-inflammatory effects of e-cigarette vapour condensate on human alveolar macrophages. Thorax. 2018;73(12):1161–9.
25. Madison MC, Landers CT, Gu BH, Chang CY, Tung HY, You R, Hong MJ, Baghaei N, Song LZ, Porter P, Putluri N, Salas R, Gilbert BE, Levental I, Campen MJ, Corry DB, Kheradmand F. Electronic cigarettes disrupt lung lipid homeostasis and innate immunity independent of nicotine. J Clin Invest. 2019;129(10):4290–304.
26. Clapp PW, Pawlak EA, Lackey JT, Keating JE, Reeber SL, Glish GL, Jaspers I. Flavored e-cigarette liquids and cinnamaldehyde impair respiratory innate immune cell function. Am J Physiol Lung Cell Mol Physiol. 2017;313(2):L278–92.
27. Baz AA, Hao H, Lan S, Li Z, Liu S, Chen S, Chu Y. Neutrophil extracellular traps in bacterial infections and evasion strategies. Front Immunol. 2024;15:1357967.
28. Reidel B, Radicioni G, Clapp PW, Ford AA, Abdelwahab S, Rebuli ME, Haridass P, Alexis NE, Jaspers I, Kesimer M. E-cigarette use causes a unique innate immune response in the lung, involving increased neutrophilic activation and altered mucin secretion. Am J Respir Crit Care Med. 2018;197(4):492–501.
29. Twaddell SH, Baines KJ, Grainge C, Gibson PG. The emerging role of neutrophil extracellular traps in respiratory disease. Chest. 2019;156(4):774–82.
30. Chatterjee S, Tao JQ, Johncola A, Guo W, Caporale A, Langham MC, Wehrli FW. Acute exposure to e-cigarettes causes inflammation and pulmonary endothelial oxidative stress in non-smoking, healthy young subjects. Am J Physiol Lung Cell Mol Physiol. 2019;317(2):L155–66.
31. Christensen CH, Chang JT, Rostron BL, et al. Biomarkers of inflammation and oxidative stress among adult former smoker, current e-cigarette users-results from wave 1 PATH study. Cancer Epidemiol Biomarkers Prev. 2021;30(10):1947–55.
32. Lim HB, Kim SH. Inhallation of e-cigarette cartridge solution aggravates allergen-induced airway inflammation and hyper-responsiveness in mice. Toxicol Res. 2014;30(1):13–8.

33. Lerner CA, Sundar IK, Yao H, Gerloff J, Ossip DJ, McIntosh S, Robinson R, Rahman I. Vapors produced by electronic cigarettes and e-juices with flavorings induce toxicity, oxidative stress, and inflammatory response in lung epithelial cells and in mouse lung. PLoS One. 2015;10(2):e0116732.
34. Husari A, Shihadeh A, Talih S, Hashem Y, El Sabban M, Zaatari G. Acute exposure to electronic and combustible cigarette aerosols: effects in an animal model and in human alveolar cells. Nicotine Tob Res. 2016;18(5):613–9.
35. Song MA, Freudenheim JL, Brasky TM, Mathe EA, McElroy JP, Nickerson QA, Reisinger SA, Smiraglia DJ, Weng DY, Ying KL, Wewers MD, Shields PG. Biomarkers of exposure and effect in the lungs of smokers, nonsmokers, and electronic cigarette users. Cancer Epidemiol Biomarkers Prev. 2020;29(2):443–51.
36. Goel R, Durand E, Trushin N, Prokopczyk B, Foulds J, Elias RJ, Richie JP Jr. Highly reactive free radicals in electronic cigarette aerosols. Chem Res Toxicol. 2015;28(9):1675–7.
37. Haddad C, Salman R, El-Hellani A, Talih S, Shihadeh A, Saliba NA. Reactive oxygen species emissions from supra-and sub-ohm electronic cigarettes. J Anal Toxicol. 2019;43(1):45–50.
38. U.S. Food and Drug Administration. Lung injuries associated with use of vaping products [Internet]. Silver Spring (MD): FDA; [updated 2020 Jan 14; cited 2025 May 15]. https://www.fda.gov/news-events/public-health-focus/lung-injuries-associated-use-vaping-products.
39. Centers for Disease Control and Prevention. Outbreak of lung injury associated with the use of e-cigarette, or vaping, products [Internet]. Atlanta (GA): CDC; [cited 2025 May 15]. https://archive.cdc.gov/www_cdc_gov/tobacco/basic_information/e-cigarettes/severe-lung-disease.html.
40. Moritz ED, Zapata LB, Lekiachvili A, et al. Update: characteristics of patients in a national outbreak of e-cigarette, or vaping, product use-associated lung injuries—United States, October 2019. MMWR Morb Mortal Wkly Rep. 2019;68(43):985–9. https://doi.org/10.15585/mmwr.mm6843e1. Erratum in: MMWR Morb Mortal Wkly Rep. 2019;68(50):1170. https://doi.org/10.15585/mmwr.mm6850a6. PMID: 31671085; PMCID: PMC6822806.
41. Siegel DA, Jatlaoui TC, Koumans EH, et al. Update: interim guidance for health care providers evaluating and caring for patients with suspected e-cigarette, or vaping, product use associated lung injury—United States, October 2019. MMWR Morb Mortal Wkly Rep. 2019;68(41):919–27. https://doi.org/10.15585/mmwr.mm6841e3. PMID: 31633675; PMCID: PMC6802682.
42. Layden JE, Ghinai I, Pray I, et al. Pulmonary illness related to e-cigarette use in Illinois and Wisconsin—final report. N Engl J Med. 2020;382(10):903–16. https://doi.org/10.1056/NEJMoa1911614. Epub 2019 Sep 6. PMID: 31491072.
43. Crotty Alexander LE, Ware LB, Calfee CS, Callahan SJ, Eissenberg T, Farver C, Goniewicz ML, Jaspers I, Kheradmand F, King TE Jr, Meyer NJ. E-cigarette or vaping product use–associated lung injury: developing a research agenda. An NIH workshop report. Am J Respir Crit Care Med. 2020;202(6):795–802.
44. Kligerman S, Raptis C, Larsen B, Henry TS, Caporale A, Tazelaar H, Schiebler ML, Wehrli FW, Klein JS, Kanne J. Radiologic, pathologic, clinical, and physiologic findings of electronic cigarette or vaping product use–associated lung injury (EVALI): evolving knowledge and remaining questions. Radiology. 2020;294(3):491–505.
45. Schier JG, Meiman JG, Layden J, et al. Severe pulmonary disease associated with electronic-cigarette-product use—interim guidance. MMWR Morb Mortal Wkly Rep. 2019;68(36):787–90. https://doi.org/10.15585/mmwr.mm6836e2. Erratum in: MMWR Morb Mortal Wkly Rep. 2019;68(38):830. https://doi.org/10.15585/mmwr.mm6838a4. PMID: 31513561; PMCID: PMC6755818.
46. Blount BC, Karwowski MP, Shields PG, et al. Vitamin E acetate in bronchoalveolar-lavage fluid associated with EVALI. N Engl J Med. 2020;382(8):697–705. https://doi.org/10.1056/NEJMoa1916433. Epub 2019 Dec 20. PMID: 31860793; PMCID: PMC7032996.
47. Chen W, Wang P, Ito K, Fowles J, Shusterman D, Jaques PA, Kumagai K. Measurement of heating coil temperature for e-cigarettes with a "top-coil" clearomizer. PLoS One. 2018;13(4):e0195925.

48. Shorr AF, Scoville SL, Cersovsky SB, Shanks GD, Ockenhouse CF, Smoak BL, Carr WW, Petruccelli BP. Acute eosinophilic pneumonia among US Military personnel deployed in or near Iraq. JAMA. 2004;292(24):2997–3005. https://doi.org/10.1001/jama.292.24.2997. PMID: 15613668.
49. Uchiyama H, Suda T, Nakamura Y, Shirai M, Gemma H, Shirai T, Toyoshima M, Imokawa S, Yasuda K, Ida M, Nakano Y, Inui N, Sato J, Hayakawa H, Chida K. Alterations in smoking habits are associated with acute eosinophilic pneumonia. Chest. 2008;133(5):1174–80. https://doi.org/10.1378/chest.07-2669. Epub 2008 Feb 8. PMID: 18263675.
50. Henry TS, Kligerman SJ, Raptis CA, Mann H, Sechrist JW, Kanne JP. Imaging findings of vaping-associated lung injury. AJR Am J Roentgenol. 2020;214(3):498–505. https://doi.org/10.2214/AJR.19.22251. Epub 2019 Oct 8. PMID: 31593518.
51. Garg I, Vidholia A, Garg A, Singh S, Agahi A, Laroia A, Saboo SS, Comellas AP, Hoffman EA, Nagpal P. E-cigarette or vaping product use-associated lung injury: a review of clinico-radio-pathological characteristics. Respir Investig. 2022;60(6):738–49. https://doi.org/10.1016/j.resinv.2022.06.011. Epub 2022 Aug 11. PMID: 35963780.
52. Saqi A, Mukhopadhyay S, Butt Y, Doxtader E, Heymann JJ, Larsen BT, Moreira AL, Patel A, Reynolds JP, Sung S, Crapanzano JP. E-cigarette or vaping product use-associated lung injury: what is the role of cytologic assessment? Cancer Cytopathol. 2020;128(6):371–80. https://doi.org/10.1002/cncy.22237. Epub 2020 Jan 27. PMID: 31985892.
53. Butt YM, Smith ML, Tazelaar HD, Vaszar LT, Swanson KL, Cecchini MJ, Boland JM, Bois MC, Boyum JH, Froemming AT, Khoor A. Pathology of vaping-associated lung injury. N Engl J Med. 2019;381(18):1780–1.
54. Mukhopadhyay S, Mehrad M, Dammert P, Arrossi AV, Sarda R, Brenner DS, Maldonado F, Choi H, Ghobrial M. Lung biopsy findings in severe pulmonary illness associated with e-cigarette use (vaping). A report of eight cases. Am J Clin Pathol. 2020;153(1):30–9.
55. De Troyer A, Estenne M. Coordination between rib cage muscles and diaphragm during quiet breathing in humans. J Appl Physiol Respir Environ Exerc Physiol. 1984;57(3):899–906.
56. Leanderson R, Sundberg J, von Euler C. Role of diaphragmatic activity during singing: a study of transdiaphragmatic pressures. J Appl Physiol (1985). 1987;62(1):259–70.
57. Traser L, Burk F, Özen AC, Burdumy M, Bock M, Blaser D, Richter B, Echternach M. Respiratory kinematics and the regulation of subglottic pressure for phonation of pitch jumps—a dynamic MRI study. PLoS One. 2020;15(12):e0244539.
58. De Troyer A, Boriek AM. Mechanics of the respiratory muscles. Compr Physiol. 2011;1(3):1273–300.
59. Salomoni S, van den Hoorn W, Hodges P. Breathing and singing: objective characterization of breathing patterns in classical singers. PLoS One. 2016;11(5):e0155084.
60. Han JN, Gayan-Ramirez G, Dekhuijzen R, Decramer M. Respiratory function of the rib cage muscles. Eur Respir J. 1993;6(5):722–8.
61. Park B, Choi HG. Association between asthma and dysphonia: a population-based study. J Asthma. 2016;53(7):679–83.
62. Dogan M, Eryuksel E, Kocak I, Celikel T, Sehitoglu MA. Subjective and objective evaluation of voice quality in patients with asthma. J Voice. 2007;21(2):224–30.
63. Hamdan AL, Ziade G, Kasti M, Akl L, Bawab I, Kanj N. Phonatory symptoms and acoustic findings in patients with asthma: a cross-sectional controlled study. Indian J Otolaryngol Head Neck Surg. 2017;69(1):42–6.
64. Lavy JA, Wood G, Rubin JS, Harries M. Dysphonia associated with inhaled steroids. J Voice. 2000;14(4):581–58.
65. Stanton AE, Sellars C, Mackenzie K, McConnachie A, Bucknall CE. Perceived vocal morbidity in a problem asthma clinic. J Laryngol Otol. 2009;123(1):96–102.
66. Rachelefsky GS, Liao Y, Faruqi R. Impact of inhaled corticosteroid-induced oropharyngeal adverse events: results from a meta-analysis. Ann Allergy Asthma Immunol. 2007;98(3):225–38.
67. Ihre E, Zetterstrom O, Ihre E, Hammarberg B. Voice problems as side effects of inhaled corticosteroids patients—a prevalence study. J Voice. 2004;18:403–14.

68. Hamdan A-L, Sataloff RT, Hawkshaw MJ. Laryngeal manifestations of respiratory disorders. In: Hamdan A-L, Sataloff RT, Hawkshaw MJ, editors. Laryngeal manifestations of systemic diseases. San Diego: Plural Publishing; 2020. p. 159–83.
69. Bassi D, Furkim AM, Silva CA, Coelho MS, Rolim MR, Alencar ML, Machado MJ. Identification of risk groups for oropharyngeal dysphagia in hospitalized patients in a university hospital. Codas. 2014;26(1):17–27. PMID: 24714855.
70. Ryu CH, Han S, Lee MS, et al. Voice changes in elderly adults: prevalence and the effect of social, behavioral, and health status on voice quality. J Am Geriatr Soc. 2015;63(8):1608–14.
71. Kozak E, Maniecka-Aleksandrowicz B, Frank-Piskorska A, Witman D. Evaluation of the effect of chronic steroid inhalation therapy on the state of the upper airway in patients with chronic obstructive pulmonary disease. Pneumonol Alergol Pol. 1991;59(9–10):33–137.

8 Oral Symptoms and Findings in E-Cigarette Users and Their Impact on Voice

The impact of e-cigarette use on the oral cavity is still under thorough investigation, with growing concerns about oral health. As the oral cavity represents the first anatomic interface with e-cigarette aerosol before reaching the lower airway, it is inevitably exposed to the reactive toxins present in the e-cigarette vapors. At high concentrations, these can be retained in the host fluids/tissues, causing damage to the host cells. As a result of the disturbance in oral homeostasis, several symptoms may arise [1–3]. In a survey on e-cigarette use that included 200 e-cigarette users, Baweja et al. noted dry mouth as the most common side effect reported by e-cigarette users. A commonly used theme was "Dry mouth occurred more when I first started using the e-cigarette, and was every time I used it" [4]. Li et al. analyzed the symptoms of e-cigarette users in relation to e-liquid components using social media posts and noted an association between the nature/severity of the symptom and the concentration of propylene glycol, vegetable glycerin, and the different flavor extracts. Throat hit, which is the feeling of smoke hitting the back of your throat, was high in those who used tobacco flavor with a high propylene glycol ratio, and high in those who used menthol flavors with a varied ratio of vegetable glycerin to propylene glycol [5].

In a systematic review on the impact of e-cigarettes on oral health, Yang et al. stratified the effects into seven categories, including mouth and throat, dental and peri-odontogenic, oncologic, traumatic, and hygiene-related [3]. In this chapter, the authors stratified the impact of e-cigarettes on oral health into four categories: impact on oral microbiome, impact on saliva, impact on oral mucosa, and impact on odontogenic and dental health.

A.-l. Hamdan, *E-Cigarette Smoking, Voice, and Health*,
https://doi.org/10.1007/978-3-032-04913-1_8

E-Cigarette, Oral Microbiome, and Voice

There are controversial reports on the effect of e-cigarette liquid and aerosol on the oral microbiome. Catala-Valentin examined the impact of e-cigarettes on oral microbia by exposing commensal *Streptococcus sanguinis* and *Streptococcus gordonii* to e-cigarette aerosol and noted a decrease in the growth of these streptococci. On the other hand, e-cigarette aerosol enhanced biofilm formation of *Streptococcus mutans* and its coaggregation. The authors noted that smoking-induced dysregulation of oral bacterial homeostasis and the increase in colonization of opportunistic bacteria can open a niche for new infections [6]. Chopyk et al. conducted an analysis of the microbial community of saliva samples of e-cigarette users and noted a higher alpha diversity and operational taxonomic units in comparison to non-smokers. The buccal mucosa swabs also exhibited a shift in beta diversity and a difference in several bacterial taxa [7]. Xu et al. conducted a study on the salivary oral microbiome of 101 periodontitis patients. Among those 101 patients, 32 of them were e-cigarette smokers. The others were conventional cigarette smokers and non-smokers. The results showed an increase in several pathogens, some of which correlated with pro-inflammatory markers such as TNF-alpha and IL-1Beta. The authors concluded that e-cigarettes can cause dysbiosis of the oral microbiome, which in turn may contribute to periodontal diseases [8]. On the other hand, Nelson et al. investigated the impact of e-cigarettes on the growth of common oral streptococci and noted little or no effect, unlike conventional smoking, which led to inhibition of streptococcus growth. The study was conducted using three strains of commensal streptococci, which were exposed to various numbers of e-cigarette aerosol puffs with and without nicotine [9]. These results concurred with those of Cuadra et al., who also tested the impact of flavorless e-cigarette-generated aerosol on the growth of four strains of commensal streptococci and noted only a modest effect on biofilms and agar colonies [10]. In another pilot study, Stewart et al. investigated the impact of e-cigarettes on the oral and gut microbiota of 10 subjects who had their buccal swabs and saliva examined using V4 16S rRNA gene sequencing. There was no significant difference in alpha or beta diversity, nor in taxonomic relative abundances in comparison to controls, unlike tobacco smoking, which showed a significant impact on the bacterial profiles. The authors concluded that e-cigarette smoking was safer than traditional smoking on oral microbiota, although larger studies are needed to further understand the effect of e-cigarette smoking on oral microbiota [11]. Using the same rRNA analysis in saliva samples of five e-cigarette smokers, Wang et al. reported that e-cigarette smoking had an effect on the oral microbiota but was different than that noted in tobacco smokers [12].

How does a change in oral microbiota affect voice? There are no studies on laryngeal microbiota in e-cigarette smokers in comparison to conventional smokers and non-smokers. However, if exposure of the vocal folds to e-cigarette aerosol leads to a change in the laryngeal microbiome, this will increase the likelihood of biofilm formation and the risk of infection, similar to what has been reported in other sites of the upper airway. The increased risk for laryngotracheal diseases can be extrapolated based on previous studies on patients with laryngeal/tracheal prosthesis and biofilms. This remains hypothetical, and future investigations are needed to elucidate the effect of e-cigarette use on laryngeal biofilm and the associated risk of voice disorders.

E-Cigarette, Saliva, and Voice

Numerous studies have shown that e-cigarettes cause an alteration in salivary flow and composition. Cichonska et al. investigated the physicochemical properties of saliva of 40 e-cigarette users and noted significant changes in salivary lysosome and lactoferrin concentrations [13]. Ye et al. examined the systemic inflammatory mediators and the salivary biological profile of e-cigarette users and found a statistically significant difference in myeloperoxidase and matrix metalloproteinase-9 compared to non-smokers. The authors stressed the adverse effect of inflammatory mediators on oral health [14]. Pushalkar et al. reported an alteration in beta-diversity and abundance of *Porphyromanis* and *Veillonella* among vapors. E-cigarette users also had elevated IL-6 and IL-1β in comparison to non-smokers [15]. Pandarathodiyil et al. reported significantly higher levels of lactate dehydrogenase enzyme activity in the saliva of e-cigarette smokers in comparison to non-smokers (35.15 ± 24.34 mU/ml vs. 21.45 ± 15.30 mU/ml, respectively). Salivary LDH enzyme activity was computed using an LDH colorimetric assay kit in a cohort of 88 subjects, 29 of whom were vapors [16]. Cichonska et al. investigated the impact of e-cigarette use on the antioxidant capacity of saliva in a cohort of 35 e-cigarette users. Their results showed a lower total antioxidant status and lower Trolox equivalent antioxidant capacity in smokers (traditional and e-cigarettes) compared to non-smokers. Moreover, e-cigarette users had a higher concentration of uric acid in comparison to non-smokers [17].

How does a reduction in salivary flow and a change in salivary composition affect voice? Saliva plays a paramount role in phonation. This premise is supported by numerous studies showing that patients with oral dryness are more likely to have voice complaints than healthy subjects. In a study on 101 patients with Sjogren Syndrome (SS), Pierce et al. noted that almost 60% had current voice disorders. Sjogren's syndrome is an autoimmune disorder that affects salivary and lacrimal glands, resulting in acinar destruction, which leads to secretory reduction and xerostomia. In that study, the authors used a self-reported outcome measure, namely a questionnaire that participants were asked to fill out [18]. The increased risk for voice complaints in patients with oral dryness can be ascribed to an alteration in vocal fold vibration during phonation. In a study on women with SS, Salturk et al. reported significant changes in vocal fold closure and smoothness in comparison to subjects with no SS [19]. In another study by Roh et al., which included 10 men with drug-induced xerostomia, the authors reported a correlation between vocal effort/change and the decrease in salivary flow [20]. Grinstein-Koren et al. reported worse auditory perceptual rating for roughness and grade of dysphonia, and higher Voice Handicap Index-10 (VHI-10) scores in 24 patients diagnosed with xerostomia. These subjective findings were associated with an increase in cycle-to-cycle variation in frequency [21]. Along the same line of investigation, many studies demonstrated that systemic dehydration during fasting also resulted in voice fatigue and an increase in phonatory effort [22–24].

All the above lead us to conclude that a reduction in salivary flow has an adverse effect on voice. There are no studies on voice characteristics of e-cigarette users with oral dryness or xerostomia; however, there are a few documenting a higher prevalence of voice complaints in e-cigarette users. The etiologic role of salivary reduction in these patients is still unknown. Future studies are needed to explore the potential role of xerostomia on the risk of voice disorders in e-cigarette users with voice disorders.

E-Cigarette, Oral Mucosa, and Voice

Numerous studies suggest the presence of a link between e-cigarette use and lesions of the oral mucosa. This is not surprising given the adverse effects of e-cigarettes on the oral microbiome and salivary function. Cho investigated the link between e-cigarette use and gingival pain/bleeding and tongue/inside cheek pain in a cross-sectional study of 65,528 students, of whom 0.5% were daily e-cigarette users and 1.9% were past-month users (1–29 days). The adjusted odds ratio (OR) for tongue/inside check pain in "daily e-cigarette users" compared to "never e-cigarette users" was 1.54 [25]. Nguyen et al. reported two cases of oral carcinoma following the use of e-cigarettes for more than 10 years. Reported symptoms included dry mouth, difficulty swallowing, and weight loss. Neither of the two patients had other risk factors for oral carcinoma, such as alcohol consumption, history of chronic oral infection, or positive family history of oral cancer. On physical examination, one patient had exophytic masses with hyperkeratosis of the tongue, biopsy of which was consistent with basaloid squamous cell carcinoma. The second patient had a lower lip ulceration at the vermillion border. Biopsy of the lesion revealed basaloid squamous cell carcinoma. The authors deliberated on the pathophysiology of these lesions in smokers with emphasis on smoking-induced decrease in salivary antioxidant capacity and the pathogenic role of the various ingredients of e-cigarettes such as nicotine, propylene glycol, and glycerin [26]. Bardellini et al. reported a higher prevalence of oral mucosal lesions in e-cigarette users ($n = 45$) (at least 6 months) in comparison to former smokers ($n = 45$). Nineteen of the former smoker group had an oral mucosal lesion vs. 36 in the e-cigarette consumer group. The authors noted the higher prevalence of hairy tongue, nicotine stomatitis, and angular cheilitis in e-cigarette users [27]. Ralho et al. conducted a systematic review of the literature on the effect of e-cigarette use on the oral cavity and reported nicotine stomatitis, angular cheilitis, and hairy tongue among the nine most common oral mucosal lesions [28]. Guo and Hecht conducted a review of the literature on e-cigarette-induced DNA damage to human oral cells. Clinical studies showed that e-cigarette users had fewer apurinic/apyrimidinic sites and higher levels of acrolein DNA adducts, metanuclear anomalies, and lactate dehydrogenase enzyme expression. In vitro studies revealed genotoxicity, DNA damage, and double-stranded breaks in addition to apoptosis and oxidative stress [29].

How do oral mucosal lesions affect the voice? The oral cavity is a main resonator in voice production. Resonance, defined as amplification of sound by the mechanism of reflection on various structures, is affected by the shape and configuration of the resonators [30–33]. Functional imaging of singers performing phonatory tasks in different vocal registers confirmed the variation in oropharyngeal and laryngeal dimensions with a change in pitch and loudness [30]. The position of the tongue and lips plays a paramount role in shaping the position and dispersion of the first two formant frequencies. Protrusion of the lips, for instance, can lower formant frequencies similar to the effect of lowering the larynx [31–34]. A low base of tongue and a high palate help in amplifying the voice by creating more depth and volume for sound projection. Singers very often modulate the shape of the laryngopharyngeal complex in an attempt to cluster the formants' energy and improve performance. Based on the above, it is fair to assume that patients with oropharyngeal lesions are more likely to have voice and swallowing complaints than healthy subjects. Indeed, there are a few reports on the voice characteristics of patients with oral lesions following chemoradiation treatment of cancer of the head and neck, asserting this hypothesis. Soldatova and Mirza investigated the long-term voice and swallowing outcomes of 28 patients with oral and oropharyngeal cancer who had primary or adjuvant chemoradiation therapy. The results showed that almost one-third (32%) had a VHI-10 and an EAT-10 score above or equal to 20. The most commonly reported vocal symptoms were lowered pitch, breathiness, and voice fatigue [35]. The authors attributed the voice and swallowing problems to mucosal erythema, fibrosis, and xerostomia, which are common acute toxicities of chemoradiation [36]. Campos et al. conducted a cross-sectional study on voice characteristics of 25 patients with head and neck cancer, including 12% with oral cavity cancer, who were treated with radiotherapy and or chemotherapy. The results showed that 40% reported hoarseness and 36% had moderate dysphonia on auditory perceptual evaluation. Moreover, close to half complained of throat clearing [37].

There are no reports in the literature on the voice characteristics of e-cigarette users with oral mucosal lesions. However, one can extrapolate from the reports on voice and swallowing disorders in patients post-chemoradiation that e-cigarette smokers with oral mucosal lesions and stomatitis are more likely to have voice and swallowing complaints than healthy subjects. Future studies on the etiologic role of oral mucosal pathology on voice in e-cigarette users are needed.

E-Cigarette, Odontogenic Health, and Voice

The use of e-cigarettes has been associated with poor periodontal and dental health. In a systematic review on the impact of e-cigarette use on the oral cavity, Ralho et al. reported worse periodontal diseases and peri-implant conditions among e-cigarette and conventional cigarette users compared to non-smokers. Non-smokers had more bleeding on probing than e-cigarette and conventional cigarette smokers

[28]. Palomino et al. conducted a study looking at the effect of e-cigarettes on dental enamel using 63 bovine enamel specimens exposed to aerosols of e-liquids of various flavors and different nicotine concentrations. Following exposure to 20 cycles, the authors noted a decrease in the luminosity of the enamel at almost all concentrations of nicotine. The color change was noticed more when flavored e-liquids were used [38]. Thiem et al. reported significantly less plaque formation or index, probing depth, marginal bone loss, and attachment loss in cigarette smokers in comparison to e-cigarette smokers. E-cigarette users had a lower risk of bleeding on probing than conventional smokers. The authors concluded that vaping is harmful but remains safer than conventional smoking regarding periodontal health [39]. In another study on clinical periodontal status of e-cigarette users, BinShabaib et al. reported a higher marginal bone loss in e-cigarette users compared to non-smokers. Moreover, non-smokers had more bleeding on probing than e-cigarette smokers and conventional cigarette smokers [40]. Ibraheem et al. conducted a prospective study that included 30 electronic-nicotine-delivery system users and noted higher scores of plaque index and probing depth compared to non-smokers [41]. Xu et al. reported worse periodontal disease in e-cigarette and cigarette smokers compared to non-smokers. In their study, which included 159 participants, the authors also noted an increase in clinical attachment loss uniquely in e-cigarette smokers ($n = 32$) [42].

The increase in dental and odontogenic diseases can be ascribed to poor oral health, as noted in the previous section of this chapter. Huilgol et al. conducted a survey that included 456,343 participants, among whom 4957 were daily e-cigarette users, and found an association between e-cigarette smoking and poor oral health. The odds of poor oral health in e-cigarette smokers were 1.78 (95% CI) [43]. Rouabhia and Semlali reported an increase in the growth of *Streptococcus mutans* (*S. mutans*) following exposure of *S. mutans* cells to e-cigarette aerosol for 15 min twice a day. The authors also noted an increase in the adherence of *S. mutans* cells to the tooth surface and an overexpression of glucan-binding genes, glucosyltransferase [44].

How does poor dental health affect the voice? Poor dental health and odontogenic diseases can impact phonation by affecting the morphology of the upper and lower jaw. In a study on the morphologic characteristics of bony edentulous jaws, Pietrokovski et al. noted centripetal maxillary resorption and centrifugal mandibular resorption after tooth loss, which affected the occlusal surfaces of the edentulous jaws [45]. In another study on mandibular jaw angle and tooth retention, Ohm and Silness reported a larger gonial angle in edentulous participants compared to those who retained their teeth. The gonial angle is the angle between the posterior and lower part of the mandible and is in the range of 100–148° [46].

As part of the phonatory apparatus, the dentofacial skeleton defines the boundaries of the oral division of the vocal tract. To that end, patients with dentofacial anomalies or alterations secondary to poor dental and periodontal health may exhibit distinct voice characteristics. There are no studies on the acoustic properties of e-cigarette users with periodontal diseases; however, there are many reports on the association between dentofacial morphology and voice. Hamdan et al. reported a negative correlation between maxillary arch depth and the third formant for vowels

/a/. /i/ and /u/, and a positive correlation with the second formant for the vowel /o/. Similarly, there was a negative correlation between the length of the maxillary arch and the fourth formant for certain vowels [47]. There are also numerous studies on the strong interplay between voice and dentoskeletal occlusion, which is impacted by dental diseases. Macari et al. reported a negative correlation between the mandibular and maxillary length and width and the third and fourth formants for given vowels. The width of the upper and lower jaws was also linked to the formant dispersion, i.e., the interspace between the formants [48].

References

1. Ebersole J, Samburova V, Son Y, Cappelli D, Demopoulos C, Capurro A, Pinto A, Chrzan B, Kingsley K, Howard K, Clark N. Harmful chemicals emitted from electronic cigarettes and potential deleterious effects in the oral cavity. Tob Induc Dis. 2020;18:41.
2. Holliday R, Chaffee BW, Jakubovics NS, Kist R, Preshaw PM. Electronic cigarettes and oral health. J Dent Res. 2021;100(9):906–13.
3. Yang I, Sandeep S, Rodriguez J. The oral health impact of electronic cigarette use: a systematic review. Crit Rev Toxicol. 2020;50(2):97–127.
4. Baweja R, Curci KM, Yingst J, Veldheer S, Hrabovsky S, Wilson SJ, Nichols TT, Eissenberg T, Foulds J. Views of experienced electronic cigarette users. Addict Res Theory. 2016;24(1):80–8.
5. Li Q, Zhan Y, Wang L, Leischow SJ, Zeng DD. Analysis of symptoms and their potential associations with e-liquids' components: a social media study. BMC Public Health. 2016;16:1–2.
6. Catala-Valentin A, Bernard JN, Caldwell M, Maxson J, Moore SD, Andl CD. E-cigarette aerosol exposure favors the growth and colonization of oral Streptococcus mutans compared to commensal streptococci. Microbiol Spectr. 2022;10(2):e02421-21.
7. Chopyk J, Bojanowski CM, Shin J, Moshensky A, Fuentes AL, Bonde SS, Chuki D, Pride DT, Crotty Alexander LE. Compositional differences in the oral microbiome of e-cigarette users. Front Microbiol. 2021;12:599664.
8. Xu F, Pushalkar S, Lin Z, Thomas SC, Persaud JK, Sierra MA, Vardhan M, Vasconcelos R, Akapo A, Guo Y, Gordon T. Electronic cigarette use enriches periodontal pathogens. Mol Oral Microbiol. 2022;37(2):63–76.
9. Nelson JM, Cuadra GA, Palazzolo DL. A comparison of flavorless electronic cigarette-generated aerosol and conventional cigarette smoke on the planktonic growth of common oral commensal streptococci. Int J Environ Res Public Health. 2019;16(24):5004.
10. Cuadra GA, Smith MT, Nelson JM, Loh EK, Palazzolo DL. A comparison of flavorless electronic cigarette-generated aerosol and conventional cigarette smoke on the survival and growth of common oral commensal streptococci. Int J Environ Res Public Health. 2019;16(10):1669.
11. Stewart CJ, Auchtung TA, Ajami NJ, Velasquez K, Smith DP, De La Garza R II, Salas R, Petrosino JF. Effects of tobacco smoke and electronic cigarette vapor exposure on the oral and gut microbiota in humans: a pilot study. PeerJ. 2018;6:e4693.
12. Wang X, Mi Q, Yang J, Guan Y, Zeng W, Xiang H, Liu X, Yang W, Yang G, Li X, Cui Y, Gao Q. Effect of electronic cigarette and tobacco smoking on the human saliva microbial community. Braz J Microbiol. 2022;53(2):991–1000. https://doi.org/10.1007/s42770-022-00721-5.
13. Cichońska D, Kusiak A, Kochańska B, Ochocińska J, Świetlik D. Influence of electronic cigarettes on selected antibacterial properties of saliva. Int J Environ Res Public Health. 2019;16(22):4433.
14. Ye D, Gajendra S, Lawyer G, Jadeja N, Pishey D, Pathagunti S, Lyons J, Veazie P, Watson G, McIntosh S, Rahman I. Inflammatory biomarkers and growth factors in saliva and gingival crevicular fluid of e-cigarette users, cigarette smokers, and dual smokers: a pilot study. J Periodontol. 2020;91(10):1274–83. https://doi.org/10.1002/JPER.19-0457.

15. Pushalkar S, Paul B, Li Q, Yang J, Vasconcelos R, Makwana S, González JM, Shah S, Xie C, Janal MN, Queiroz E. Electronic cigarette aerosol modulates the oral microbiome and increases risk of infection. Iscience. 2020;23(3):100884.
16. Pandarathodiyil AK, Ramanathan A, Garg R, Doss JG, Abd Rahman FB, Ghani WM, Warnakulasuriya S. Lactate dehydrogenase levels in the saliva of cigarette and E-cigarette smokers (vapers): a comparative analysis. Asian Pac J Cancer Prev APJCP. 2021;22(10):3227.
17. Cichońska D, Król O, Słomińska EM, Kochańska B, Świetlik D, Ochocińska J, Kusiak A. Influence of electronic cigarettes on antioxidant capacity and nucleotide metabolites in saliva. Toxics. 2021;9(10):263.
18. Pierce JL, Tanner K, Merrill RM, Miller KL, Ambati BK, Kendall KA, Roy N. Voice disorders in Sjögren's syndrome: prevalence and related risk factors. Laryngoscope. 2015;125(6):1385–92.
19. Saltürk Z, Özdemir E, Kumral TL, Karabacakoğlu Z, Kumral E, Yildiz HE, Mersinlioğlu G, Atar Y, Berkiten G, Yildirim G, Uyar Y. Subjective and objective voice evaluation in Sjögren's syndrome. Logoped Phoniatr Vocol. 2017;42(1):9–11.
20. Roh JL, Kim HS, Kim AY. The effect of acute xerostomia on vocal function. Arch Otolaryngol Head Neck Surg. 2006;132(5):542–6.
21. Grinstein-Koren O, Herzog N, Amir O. Hyposalivation affecting womens' voice. J Voice. 2023;37(3):469–e19.
22. Hamdan AL, Nassar J, Dowli A, Al Zaghal Z, Sibai A. Electroglottography in fasting subjects. J Voice. 2015;29(2):165–9. https://doi.org/10.1016/j.jvoice.2013.04.006. Epub 2015 Jan 22. PMID: 25619473.
23. Hamdan AL, Ashkar J, Sibai A, Oubari D, Husseini ST. Effect of fasting on voice in males. Am J Otolaryngol. 2011;32(2):124–9. https://doi.org/10.1016/j.amjoto.2009.12.001. Epub 2010 Apr 13. PMID: 20392525.
24. Hamdan AL, Sibai A, Rameh C. Effect of fasting on voice in women. J Voice. 2007;21(4):495–501. https://doi.org/10.1016/j.jvoice.2006.01.009. Epub 2006 Apr 19. PMID: 16630706.
25. Cho JH. The association between electronic-cigarette use and self-reported oral symptoms including cracked or broken teeth and tongue and/or inside-cheek pain among adolescents: a cross-sectional study. PLoS One. 2017;12(7):e0180506.
26. Nguyen H, Kitzmiller JP, Nguyen KT, Nguyen C, Bui T. Oral carcinoma associated with chronic use of electronic cigarettes. Otolaryngol (Sunnyvale). 2017;7(2):304.
27. Bardellini E, Amadori F, Conti G, Majorana A. Oral mucosal lesions in electronic cigarettes consumers versus former smokers. Acta Odontol Scand. 2018;76(3):226–8. https://doi.org/10.1080/00016357.2017.1406613. Epub 2017 Nov 21. PMID: 29161938.
28. Ralho A, Coelho A, Ribeiro M, Paula A, Amaro I, Sousa J, Marto C, Ferreira M, Carrilho E. Effects of electronic cigarettes on oral cavity: a systematic review. J Evid Based Dent Pract. 2019;19(4):101318.
29. Guo J, Hecht SS. DNA damage in human oral cells induced by use of e-cigarettes. Drug Test Anal. 2023;15(10):1189–97.
30. Echternach M, Burk F, Burdumy M, Traser L, Richter B. Morphometric differences of vocal tract articulators in different loudness conditions in singing. PLoS One. 2016;11(4):e0153792.
31. Macari AT, Ziade G, Khandakji M, Tamim H, Hamdan AL. Effect of rapid maxillary expansion on voice. J Voice. 2016;30(6):760–e1.
32. Marunick MT, Menaldi CJ. Maxillary dental arch form related to voice classification: a pilot study. J Voice. 2000;14(1):82–91.
33. Macari AT, Karam IA, Tabri D, Sarieddine D, Hamdan AL. Correlation between the length and sagittal projection of the upper and lower jaw and the fundamental frequency. J Voice. 2014;28(3):291–6.
34. Roers F, Mürbe D, Sundberg J. Voice classification and vocal tract of singers: a study of x-ray images and morphology. J Acoust Soc Am. 2009;125(1):503–12.
35. Soldatova L, Mirza N. Long-term voice and swallowing outcomes for oral and oropharyngeal cancer following primary or adjuvant chemoradiation. Ann Otol Rhinol Laryngol. 2019;128(9):802–10.

36. Parsons A, Dewan K. Dysphagia and dysphonia after head and neck cancer. Oral Dis. 2024.
37. Campos RJ, Maciel CT, Cesca MG, Leite IC. Voice analysis after cancer treatment with organ preservation. Head Neck Oncol. 2011;3:1–5.
38. Pintado-Palomino K, de Almeida CV, Oliveira-Santos C, Pires-de-Souza FP, Tirapelli C. The effect of electronic cigarettes on dental enamel color. J Esthet Restor Dent. 2019;31(2):160–5.
39. Thiem DG, Donkiewicz P, Rejaey R, Wiesmann-Imilowski N, Deschner J, Al-Nawas B, Kämmerer PW. The impact of electronic and conventional cigarettes on periodontal health—a systematic review and meta-analysis. Clin Oral Investig. 2023;27(9):4911–28.
40. BinShabaib M, ALHarthi SS, Akram Z, Khan J, Rahman I, Romanos GE, Javed F. Clinical periodontal status and gingival crevicular fluid cytokine profile among cigarette-smokers, electronic-cigarette users and never-smokers. Arch Oral Biol. 2019;102:212–7. https://doi.org/10.1016/j.archoralbio.2019.05.001. Epub 2019 May 3. PMID: 31078071.
41. Ibraheem WI, Fageeh HI, Preethanath RS, Alzahrani FA, Al-Zawawi AS, Divakar DD, Al-Kheraif AA. Comparison of RANKL and osteoprotegerin levels in the gingival crevicular fluid of young cigarette- and waterpipe-smokers and individuals using electronic nicotine delivery systems. Arch Oral Biol. 2020;115:104714. https://doi.org/10.1016/j.archoralbio.2020.104714. Epub 2020 Apr 11. PMID: 32442729.
42. Xu F, Aboseria E, Janal MN, Pushalkar S, Bederoff MV, Vasconcelos R, Sapru S, Paul B, Queiroz E, Makwana S, Solarewicz J, Guo Y, Aguallo D, Gomez C, Shelly D, Aphinyanaphongs Y, Gordon T, Corby PM, Kamer AR, Li X, Saxena D. Comparative effects of e-cigarette aerosol on periodontium of periodontitis patients. Front Oral Health. 2021;2:729144. https://doi.org/10.3389/froh.2021.729144. PMID: 35048050; PMCID: PMC8757783.
43. Huilgol P, Bhatt SP, Biligowda N, Wright NC, Wells JM. Association of e-cigarette use with oral health: a population-based cross-sectional questionnaire study. J Public Health. 2019;41(2):354–61.
44. Rouabhia M, Semlali A. Electronic cigarette vapor increases Streptococcus mutans growth, adhesion, biofilm formation, and expression of the biofilm-associated genes. Oral Dis. 2021;27(3):639–47.
45. Pietrokovski J, Starinsky R, Arensburg B, Kaffe I. Morphologic characteristics of bony edentulous jaws. J Prosthodont. 2007;16(2):141–7. https://doi.org/10.1111/j.1532-849X.2007.00165.x. PMID: 17362425.
46. Ohm E, Silness J. Size of the mandibular jaw angle related to age, tooth retention and gender. J Oral Rehabil. 1999;26(11):883–91. https://doi.org/10.1046/j.1365-2842.1999.00464.x. PMID: 10583739.
47. Hamdan AL, Khandakji M, Macari AT. Maxillary arch dimensions associated with acoustic parameters in prepubertal children. Angle Orthod. 2018;88(4):410–5.
48. Macari AT, Karam IA, Tabri D, Sarieddine D, Hamdan AL. Formants frequency and dispersion in relation to the length and projection of the upper and lower jaws. J Voice. 2015;29(1):83–90.

Vaping, Sinonasal Diseases, and Voice

9

Impact of E-Cigarette Smoking on the Nose and Paranasal Sinuses

The upper respiratory system, particularly the nose, acts as a first line of defense against inhaled respiratory pathogens and allergens. Following exposure to any occupational or environmental irritant, the immune system is activated and inflammatory markers are produced in an attempt to maintain homeostasis of the nasal cavity and paranasal sinuses [1]. E-cigarettes have been proven to produce several cytotoxic substances and oxidants that may be harmful to the mucosal lining of the upper respiratory system, including the nose and sinuses [2]. Numerous studies in the literature indicate that e-cigarette users are at a higher risk of developing sinonasal symptoms. Kumral et al. conducted a study on sinonasal symptoms in smokers who used e-cigarettes vs. those who used other therapeutic methods to stop smoking (referred to as non-e-cigarette smokers). Prior to cessation of smoking, there was no significant difference in the SNOT-22 score between the two groups ($p = 0.133$). After 3 months of cessation of smoking, there was a decrease in the mean SNOT-22 scores in both groups; however, the decrease was more significant in the non-e-cigarette smokers in comparison to e-cigarette smokers (17.37 ± 2.75 vs. 24.19 ± 4.49, respectively) [3]. Pingree et al. conducted a study on the effect of e-cigarette and conventional cigarette use on chronic rhinosinusitis using the TriNetX Global Collaborative Network database. The authors found that conventional cigarette users had a higher relative risk (RR) and odds ratio (OR) for chronic rhinosinusitis than e-cigarette users (1.12 and 1.13, respectively). Dual users had a higher RR and odds ratio (OR) for diagnosis of chronic rhinosinusitis and for functional endoscopic sinus surgery compared to e-cigarette users [4]. Rha et al. analyzed the data from the Korean National Health and Nutritional Examination Survey, looking for the link between e-cigarette smoking, chronic rhinosinusitis (CRS), and allergic rhinitis (AR). Among the 38,413 participants, 2.5% and 6.4% were current and former e-cigarette smokers, respectively. Logistic regression analysis while

A.-l. Hamdan, *E-Cigarette Smoking, Voice, and Health*,
https://doi.org/10.1007/978-3-032-04913-1_9

adjusting for confounders revealed higher OR for CRS among former and current e-cigarette smokers in comparison to non-e-cigarette smokers (OR = 1.35 and OR = 1.08, respectively). Similarly, former and current e-cigarette smokers had a higher odds ratio for AR than non-e-cigarette smokers (OR = 1.12 and OR = 1.43, respectively). The authors concluded that e-cigarette use is associated with a high prevalence of AR and CRS, and hence can increase the likelihood of developing diseases of the upper respiratory system [5]. Chung et al. investigated the relation between cigarette smoking (including e-cigarettes), AR, and asthma using the large survey data on Korean middle and high school students. The results showed an association between e-cigarette use and AR. Moreover, the OR for asthma was higher among individuals who used e-cigarettes and/or heated tobacco products in combination with conventional cigarettes, compared to those who had never used heated tobacco products or e-cigarettes but were current conventional cigarette smokers. The authors concluded that the use of e-cigarettes and heated product tobacco may exacerbate the negative effect of CC on AR and asthma [6]. On the other hand, in a large study by Li et al. on the link between symptoms and the ingredients of e-cigarette liquid, the authors noted that most sinus symptoms reported by e-cigarette users were positive. They have reported clearing or opening of their sinuses following e-cigarette smoking [7].

How Does E-Cigarette Increase the Risk for CRS?

The higher prevalence of CRS in e-cigarette smokers compared to non-smokers can be ascribed to several factors, most important of which is smoke-induced inflammation and altered immune response. Hwang et al. reported a dose-dependent death of human epithelial cells following exposure to fresh e-cigarette vapor (at the air–liquid interface) and a decrease in neutrophil and macrophage antimicrobial activity. Exposure of mice to e-cigarette vapor 1 h a day for 4 weeks led to immunomodulation of cytokines and inflammatory markers. The authors concluded that e-cigarette smoking promotes inflammation of the airway and alters the host defense, thus leading to more colonization of bacteria and biofilm formation [8]. Martin et al. conducted a study on the impact of e-cigarette smoking on immune-related gene expression in the nose and noted a decrease in many genes that usually decrease in conventional smoking. They also noted suppression of other unique genes ($n = 305$). The gene analysis was done on nasal scrape biopsies and nasal lavage using the Counter Human Immunology v2 Expression panel. The authors concluded that e-cigarettes, at least at the level of the nasal mucosa, can lead to immune suppression [9]. These studies concur with similar studies on the lower airway. Sussan et al. conducted an animal study and noted that exposure to e-cigarette vapor for 2 weeks can lead to inflammatory changes and oxidative stress, resulting in impairment in pulmonary bacterial clearance, which jeopardizes pulmonary defenses [10]. Ghosh et al. investigated the impact of vaping on pulmonary epithelial cells and found an alteration in several proteins commonly affected in cigarette smokers, and many others affected only in e-cigarette users, among which were the MUC5AC and

MUC4. These alterations were accompanied by visible changes in the mucosa, which became inflamed and friable. The authors also noted that membrane fluidity and protein diffusion were affected by the propylene glycol/vegetable glycerin ingredients of e-cigarette aerosol [11].

Impact of Sinonasal Diseases on Voice

There are no studies in the literature on voice characteristics of e-cigarette smokers with sinonasal diseases in comparison to e-cigarette smokers with no sinonasal diseases. However, there is a consensus that patients with sinonasal disease are at a higher risk of having voice disorders than healthy normal subjects. Several investigators showed that patients with AR and or CRS are more likely to have a high voice handicap index score and poor auditory perceptual rating. In 2008, Millqvist et al. investigated vocal dysfunction in 30 patients with well-documented birch pollen allergy and noted high VHI scores and vocal symptoms during the pollen season. The VHI-10 score of those with allergy was higher than that of those without allergy during and outside the pollen season (18.3 vs. 2.8, respectively, and 13.9 vs.6.0, respectively) [12]. In 2017, Arslan et al. conducted a study on self-perceived voice quality in 63 patients with nasal polyposis undergoing surgical treatment. The mean VHI-10 and nasalance scores preoperatively were 10.47 ± 4.81 and 8.38 ± 0.94, respectively. Both scores decreased after surgical intervention. The authors concluded that nasal obstruction has an adverse effect on voice and that surgery can help improve phonatory symptoms. They also highlighted the need to inform patients about the potential change in voice quality postoperatively [13]. In 2019, Jandali et al. investigated the effects of endoscopic sinus surgery on voice characteristics of 18 patients with chronic rhinosinusitis and noted a preoperative mean VHI-10 score of 10.2 ± 2.2, and a mean CAPE-V of 45 ± 5.9. The decrease in these scores postoperatively correlated with a decrease in the SNOT-22 score [14]. In 2019, in another study on the impact of endoscopic sinus surgeries on voice, Wong et al. found that almost one out of three (30%) patients with polyposis and 40% of their friends or relatives noticed a change in their voice preoperatively [15]. In 2016, in a cohort of 50 patients with CRS and nasal polyposis undergoing surgery, Hall et al. noted a preoperative mean VHI-10 score of 17.1 [16]. In 2020, in another study on the effect of functional endoscopic sinus surgery on Voice and Speech Recognition, which included 53 patients, 26 of whom with CRSwNP and 27 controls without nasal obstruction, Hernández-García E et al. reported a preoperative mean GRBAS of 2.15 ± 1.25 in comparison to 0.63 ± 1.08 in controls [17].

What further substantiates the adverse effect of sinus diseases on voice is the improvement in many acoustic parameters in addition to the improvement in self-reported voice symptoms following endoscopic sinus surgery. In 2014, Acar et al. performed acoustic analysis before and 6 weeks after endoscopic sinus surgery in 43 patients with different stages of nasal polyposis. Although the mean values of jitter, shimmer, and NHR varied preoperatively with the stage of the disease (Jitter 0.68 ± 0.4 to 0.9 ± 0.8, shimmer 3.46 ± 1.1 to 5.7 ± 3.1, and NHR 0.125 ± 0.008 to

0.14 ± 0.02), there was a significant decrease in the perturbation parameters and a significant increase in the fundamental frequency following surgery in patients with partial nasal obstruction. The authors stressed the need to highlight the possible changes in voice quality to patients with sinus disease undergoing sinus surgery [18]. In 2016, Atan et al. analyzed the voice characteristics of 43 patients with septal deviation undergoing septoplasty before and 1 month after surgery. The study group was divided into two subgroups: those with complete nasal obstruction (group A) and those with less severe obstruction (group B). The authors found an improvement in the VHI-30 score in both subgroups, and the improvement was significant in group B. The mean VHI-30 in group A decreased from 1.38 ± 1.98 to 0.69 ± 1.31 postoperatively, and the mean VHI-30 score for group B decreased from 1.60 ± 2.04 to 0.70 ± 1.5. Group A had improvement in all voice parameters, with a non-significant decrease in shimmer by 0.16 ($p = 0.071$) and a significant increase in F0 by 15.31 Hz ($p < 0.001$) [19]. In 2016, Gulec et al. investigated the effect of septoplasty on voice in 50 patients using subjective and objective voice measures. The authors noted that almost one out of three patients reported improvement in voice quality after surgery. Interestingly, there was no significant change in any of the acoustic parameters postoperatively [20].

Pathophysiology of Voice Disorders in Patients with Sinonasal Diseases

The pathophysiology of dysphonia in patients with sinonasal diseases is complex. Several mechanisms have been suggested; one is repetitive throat clearing. Throat clearing is a phono-traumatic behavior that leads to an increase in the collision force between the vocal folds. In a review on the stress of phonation, Titz et al. noted that the stress of collision is a mechanical stress among others, such as shearing stress, tensile stress, and aerodynamic stress [21]. With an increase in the collision force, there is an increase in intra-capillary pressure, often associated with bleeding and inflammatory changes. Czerwonka et al. reported a correlation between vocal fold vibration amplitude and frequency and capillary pressure. An increase in capillary pressure that exceeds 20 cm H_2O may elicit inflammation and injury to the vocal folds [22]. All these factors act in concert, resulting in a change in the landscape of the extracellular matrix constituents and possible mass formation. Another suggested mechanism for the change in voice quality in patients with sinus disease is laryngeal desiccation. Nasal obstruction and mouth breathing are common symptoms in patients with chronic rhinosinusitis [23–25]. Mouth breathing may lead to desiccation of the vocal tract and thinning of the vocal fold's sol layer [26, 27]. This in turn increases the phonatory threshold pressure (PTP), i.e., the pressure needed to set the vocal folds in vibration. An increase in PTP is associated with an increase in effort to talk. Sivasankar et al. investigated the impact of mouth breathing on voice and noted that mouth breathing while reading aloud or exercising increased the PTP. The increase was present in both low and high humidity environments. The study included 63 participants who had their PTP and perceived phonatory effort measured before and 15 min after mouth breathing [28]. The impact of dehydration on voice has also been asserted by studies on fasting and voice. Hamdan et al. conducted a study on the impact of fasting on voice in a cohort of 28 women and noted a higher prevalence of voice fatigue with a decrease in maximum phonation time while fasting in comparison to non-fasting [29]. Fasting consisted of abstinence from water intake for 14–18 h, which is commensurate with almost 1 L of water loss [29]. A similar study done on men also showed that systemic dehydration leads to vocal fatigue [30]. A third suggested mechanism for the link between sinus diseases and voice disorders is reflux disease. In a systematic review that included 17 studies, Lechien et al. noted the prevalence of gastroesophageal reflux disease in 32–91% of patients with CRS. Moreover, close to half of patients with recalcitrant CRS had hypo or nasopharyngeal acid reflux events. The authors concluded that reflux disease could contribute to the pathogenesis of CRS in patients who are refractory to treatment [31]. In another review on the link between reflux disease and CRS, Aldajani et al. reported a significant association between GERD and CRS. Patients with CRS exhibited higher values of pepsin in comparison to healthy controls. The strong link between reflux and sinus disease was further substantiated by the high response to proton pump inhibitors and the improvement in disease outcome following anti-reflux therapy [32]. Reflux is a known predisposing factor for functional and structural voice disorders. In a review of 150 patients diagnosed with muscle tension dysphonia, Altman et al. reported the prevalence of gastroesophageal reflux disease in 49% of the cases. The authors stressed the etiologic role of reflux disease among other factors, such as stress and high vocal load in patients with MTD [33]. In a review on the role of laryngopharyngeal reflux disease in the development of benign vocal fold lesions, Lechien et al. noted that caustic-induced injury increases the susceptibility of the vocal folds. Suggested mechanisms include alteration in cell-to-cell dehiscence and other mucosal defense mechanisms [31]. Last but not least, dysphonia in patients with CRS may be secondary to mental disorders, which range in frequency between 9% and 26% of the cases [34]. Erskine et al. investigated factors that can affect the onset and severity of CRS using a questionnaire (SF-36) in 30 centers in the United Kingdom. The results showed a higher prevalence of anxiety and depression in comparison to healthy controls. The OR for those with CRS and those without nasal polyposis was 1.40 and 1.89, respectively. The authors highlighted the need to address mental illnesses as a significant morbidity in affected patients [35]. Smith and Alt examined the link between CRS and comorbid depression and noted that 40% of patients may be underdiagnosed if not screened properly. Other precipitating factors for depression in patients with CRS and without polyps included pain, sleep disorders, and olfactory dysfunction [34]. Using population-based insurance data, which included 48,672 individuals, Kim et al. noted a higher prevalence of depression and anxiety in patients with CRS in comparison to those with no CRS. The adjusted HRs for depression and anxiety were 1.54 and 1.57, respectively. Patients with CRS without nasal polyps were at a higher risk in comparison to those with nasal polyps [36]. Wasan et al. investigated the effect of psychiatric comorbidity on disease severity in a prospective study, which included 143 patients evaluated for CRS using the Rhinosinusitis Symptom

Inventory. The results indicated that those with anxiety, depression, or combined had a higher prevalence of oropharyngeal symptoms in comparison to those without psychiatric comorbidity. The prevalence of moderate–severe anxiety and depression was 51.8% and 23.8%, respectively [37].

Mental disorders are known to affect the voice. Patients with anxiety and depression exhibit different voice characteristics than healthy subjects with no mental disorders. In a study on the correlation between anxiety, depression, and self-perceived vocal handicap, which included 620 patients with benign dysphonia, Enin et al. noted that those with anxiety and depression had worse VHI-10 scores than those without. The prevalence of anxiety and depression was 20% and 10%, respectively [38]. In another study on the ability to detect anxiety and depression using the emotional domain of the VoiSS questionnaire in comparison to the Anxiety and Depression Scale (HADS), Montgomery et al. reported mean HADS anxiety and depression of 6.5/21 and 7.1/21, respectively. Their study included 177 patients with voice disorders [39]. Elam et al. reported a correlation between the Beck Depression Inventory Fast Screen score and the VHI emotional domain in a cohort of 36 patients with laryngopharyngeal reflux and 53 controls [40].

References

1. Czerwaty K, Piszczatowska K, Brzost J, Ludwig N, Szczepański MJ, Dżaman K. Immunological aspects of chronic rhinosinusitis. Diagnostics (Basel). 2022;12(10):2361. https://doi.org/10.3390/diagnostics12102361. PMID: 36292050; PMCID: PMC9600442.
2. Lerner CA, Sundar IK, Watson RM, Elder A, Jones R, Done D, Kurtzman R, Ossip DJ, Robinson R, McIntosh S, Rahman I. Environmental health hazards of e-cigarettes and their components: oxidants and copper in e-cigarette aerosols. Environ Pollut. 2015;198:100–7.
3. Kumral TL, Saltürk Z, Yildirim G, Uyar Y, Berkiten G, Atar Y, Inan M. How does electronic cigarette smoking affect sinonasal symptoms and nasal mucociliary clearance? B-ENT. 2016;12(1):17–21.
4. Pingree G, DeShazo J, Schuman T. Impact of dual electronic and conventional cigarette use on diagnosis and surgery for chronic rhinosinusitis: a multicenter study. Int Forum Allergy Rhinol. 2024;14(5):977–80.
5. Rha MS, Cho HJ, Yoon JH, Kim CH. Association between the use of electronic cigarettes and the prevalence of chronic rhinosinusitis and allergic rhinitis: a nationwide cross-sectional study. Rhinology. 2022;60(1):20–8.
6. Chung SJ, Kim BK, Oh JH, Shim JS, Chang YS, Cho SH, Yang MS. Novel tobacco products including electronic cigarette and heated tobacco products increase risk of allergic rhinitis and asthma in adolescents: analysis of Korean youth survey. Allergy. 2020;75(7):1640–8.
7. Li Q, Zhan Y, Wang L, Leischow SJ, Zeng DD. Analysis of symptoms and their potential associations with e-liquids' components: a social media study. BMC Public Health. 2016;16:674. https://doi.org/10.1186/s12889-016-3326-0. PMID: 27475060; PMCID: PMC4967297.
8. Hwang JH, Lyes M, Sladewski K, Enany S, McEachern E, Mathew DP, Das S, Moshensky A, Bapat S, Pride DT, Ongkeko WM, Crotty Alexander LE. Electronic cigarette inhalation alters innate immunity and airway cytokines while increasing the virulence of colonizing bacteria. J Mol Med (Berl). 2016;94(6):667–79.
9. Martin EM, Clapp PW, Rebuli ME, Pawlak EA, Glista-Baker E, Benowitz NL, Fry RC, Jaspers I. E-cigarette use results in suppression of immune and inflammatory-response genes

in nasal epithelial cells similar to cigarette smoke. Am J Physiol Lung Cell Mol Physiol. 2016;311(1):L135–44.
10. Sussan TE, Gajghate S, Thimmulappa RK, Ma J, Kim JH, Sudini K, Consolini N, Cormier SA, Lomnicki S, Hasan F, Pekosz A. Exposure to electronic cigarettes impairs pulmonary anti-bacterial and anti-viral defenses in a mouse model. PLoS One. 2015;10(2):e0116861.
11. Ghosh A, Coakley RC, Mascenik T, Rowell TR, Davis ES, Rogers K, Webster MJ, Dang H, Herring LE, Sassano MF, Livraghi-Butrico A, Van Buren SK, Graves LM, Herman MA, Randell SH, Alexis NE, Tarran R. Chronic e-cigarette exposure alters the human bronchial epithelial proteome. Am J Respir Crit Care Med. 2018;198(1):67–76.
12. Millqvist E, Bende M, Brynnel M, Johansson I, Kappel S, Ohlsson AC. Voice change in seasonal allergic rhinitis. J Voice. 2008;22(4):512–5.
13. Arslan F, Polat B, Durmaz A, Birkent H. Effects of nasal obstruction due to nasal polyposis on nasal resonance and voice perception. Folia Phoniatr Logop. 2017;68(3):141–3.
14. Jandali DB, Ganti A, Husain IA, Batra PS, Tajudeen BA. The effects of endoscopic sinus surgery on voice characteristics in chronic rhinosinusitis patients. Ann Otol Rhinol Laryngol. 2019;128(12):1129–33.
15. Wong EH, Chong AW. Objective and subjective changes in voice after endoscopic sinus surgeries in patients with and without nasal polyps. Am J Otolaryngol. 2020;41(2):102367.
16. Hall CA, Hernandez SC, Barry RA, Zito BA, McWhorter AJ, Fink DS, Barham HP. Voice outcomes after endoscopic sinus surgery in patients with chronic rhinosinusitis with nasal polyposis. Laryngoscope. 2019;129(2):299–302.
17. Hernández-García E, Moro-Velázquez L, González-Herranz R, Godino-Llorente JI, Plaza G. Effect of functional endoscopic sinus surgery on voice and speech recognition. J Voice. 2020;34(4):650–e1.
18. Acar A, Cayonu M, Ozman M, Eryilmaz A. Changes in acoustic parameters of voice after endoscopic sinus surgery in patients with nasal polyposis. Indian J Otolaryngol Head Neck Surg. 2014;66:381–5.
19. Atan D, Özcan KM, Gürbüz AB, Dere H. The effect of septoplasty on voice performance in patients with severe and mild nasal septal deviation. J Craniofac Surg. 2016;27(5):1162–4.
20. Gulec S, Kulahli I, Sahin MI, Kokoğlu K, Gunes MS, Avci D, Arli T. Effect of septoplasty on voice quality: a prospective-controlled trial. Clin Exp Otorhinolaryngol. 2016;9(3):238–43.
21. Titze IR. Mechanical stress in phonation. J Voice. 1994;8(2):99–105.
22. Czerwonka L, Jiang JJ, Tao C. Vocal nodules and edema may be due to vibration-induced rises in capillary pressure. Laryngoscope. 2008;118(4):748–52.
23. Stewart M, Ferguson B, Fromer L. Epidemiology and burden of nasal congestion. Int J Gen Med. 2010;3:37–45.
24. Ferrand PA, Mercier CH, Jankowski R, Giroud C, Pasquier C, Touron D, Oriol V, Barbaza MO, Dellamonica P. Sinusites aiguës de l'adulte. Prise en charge par les médecins généralistes [Acute sinusitus in adults. Management by general practitioners]. Presse Med. 2001;30(21):1049–54.
25. Pessey JJ, Reitz C, Los F. Rhinosinusites aiguës de l'adulte: enquête nationale sur les pratiques en médecine générale [Acute rhinosinusitis in the adult: national survey of general practice management]. Rev Laryngol Otol Rhinol (Bord). 2000;121(4):237–41.
26. Sivasankar M, Leydon C. The role of hydration in vocal fold physiology. Curr Opin Otolaryngol Head Neck Surg. 2010;18(3):171–5.
27. Sivasankar M, Fisher KV. Oral breathing challenge in participants with vocal attrition. J Speech Lang Hear Res. 2003;46(6):1416–27.
28. Sivasankar MP, Erickson-Levendoski E. Influence of obligatory mouth breathing, during realistic activities, on voice measures. J Voice. 2012;26(6):813.e9–13.
29. Hamdan AL, Sibai A, Rameh C. Effect of fasting on voice in women. J Voice. 2007;21(4):495–501.
30. Hamdan AL, Ashkar J, Sibai A, Oubari D, Husseini ST. Effect of fasting on voice in males. Am J Otolaryngol. 2011;32(2):124–9.

31. Lechien JR, Saussez S, Hopkins C. Association between laryngopharyngeal reflux, gastroesophageal reflux and recalcitrant chronic rhinosinusitis: a systematic review. Clin Otolaryngol. 2023;48(4):501–14.
32. Aldajani A, Alhussain F, Mesallam T, AbaAlkhail M, Alojayri R, Bassam H, Alotaibi O, Alqahtani M, Alsaleh S. Association between chronic rhinosinusitis and reflux diseases in adults: a systematic review and meta-analysis. Am J Rhinol Allergy. 2024;38(1):47–59.
33. Altman KW, Atkinson C, Lazarus C. Current and emerging concepts in muscle tension dysphonia: a 30-month review. J Voice. 2005;19(2):261–7.
34. Smith KA, Alt JA. The relationship of chronic rhinosinusitis and depression. Curr Opin Otolaryngol Head Neck Surg. 2020;28(1):1–5.
35. Erskine SE, Hopkins C, Clark A, Anari S, Robertson A, Sunkaraneni S, Wilson JA, Beezhold J, Philpott CM. Chronic rhinosinusitis and mood disturbance. Rhinology. 2017;55(2):113–9.
36. Kim JY, Ko I, Kim MS, Yu MS, Cho BJ, Kim DK. Association of chronic rhinosinusitis with depression and anxiety in a nationwide insurance population. JAMA Otolaryngol Head Neck Surg. 2019;145(4):313–9.
37. Wasan A, Fernandez E, Jamison RN, Bhattacharyya N. Association of anxiety and depression with reported disease severity in patients undergoing evaluation for chronic rhinosinusitis. Ann Otol Rhinol Laryngol. 2007;116(7):491–7.
38. Enin K, Parikh A, Kallogjeri D, Naunheim MR, Huston MN. Correlation between a diagnosis of anxiety or depression and initial VHI-10 scores in benign dysphonia. Otolaryngol Head Neck Surg. 2022;167(4):725–30.
39. Montgomery J, Hendry J, Wilson JA, Deary IJ, MacKenzie K. Pragmatic detection of anxiety and depression in a prospective cohort of voice outpatient clinic attenders. Clin Otolaryngol. 2016;41(1):2–7.
40. Elam JC, Ishman SL, Dunbar KB, Clarke JO, Gourin CG. The relationship between depressive symptoms and Voice Handicap Index scores in laryngopharyngeal reflux. Laryngoscope. 2010;120(9):1900–3.

10 Gastrointestinal Disorders in E-Cigarette Users and Their Impact on Voice

Vaping and Gastrointestinal Disorders

The health risks of e-cigarettes are numerous, spanning every system in the body, including the gastrointestinal system. There are many studies suggesting that e-cigarette smoking, similar to combustible cigarette smoking, can precipitate esophageal and gastrointestinal disorders. In 2016, Li et al. reported stomach ache and heartburn as common digestive complaints in e-cigarette users. Based on their social media data, the authors also noted variation in symptoms with changes in the ratio of propylene glycol to vegetable glycerin [1]. In 2024, Farooqi et al. conducted a cross-sectional study on the prevalence of gastroesophageal reflux disease (GERD) in 403 students, 43% of whom were e-cigarette users. Using a validated Gastroesophageal Reflux Disease Questionnaire, the authors noted a higher score in e-cigarette users and smokers in comparison to non-smokers. Moreover, there was a relation between the frequency of vaping and symptoms of GERD [2].

The link between e-cigarettes and GI disorders has been further substantiated by many case reports describing adverse GI events following vaping. In 2014, Camus et al. reported a 49-year-old woman, a known case of ulcerative colitis (UC) refractory to medical treatment, who had complete remission and mucosal healing 1 year after resuming cigarette smoking. When this latter was replaced by e-cigarettes, 30 mg of nicotine per day, she had a relapse of her condition [3]. In 2021, Pasricha and Kochar reported a 25-year-old male patient who presented with progressive odynophagia after using e-cigarettes containing nicotine and tetrahydrocannabinol. Esophagogastroduodenoscopy revealed esophagitis involving more than one mucosal bridge. Esophageal biopsies taken showed evidence of chronic inflammation, while immunohistochemical staining for cytomegalovirus and herpes simplex was negative. The patient was managed successfully with proton pump inhibitors and analgesics [4]. In 2023, Pace and McCoogan reported a 17-year-old male patient who presented to the emergency room with throat pain, dysphagia, and odynophagia. His symptoms progressed and were associated with fever and poor tolerance to

A.-l. Hamdan, *E-Cigarette Smoking, Voice, and Health*,
https://doi.org/10.1007/978-3-032-04913-1_10

food intake. The patient had a history of vaping more than once daily. On examination, he had edema and erythema of the pharyngeal mucosa and palate associated with cervical lymphadenopathy. Esophagogastroduodenoscopy revealed esophagitis and circumferential erosion of the esophageal mucosa. Histopathologic examination and immunohistochemistry stains were not suggestive of a viral infection. The patient was hospitalized and treated with a course of antibiotics, proton pump inhibitors, and bismuth subsalicylate, which led to improvement on day 6 and complete resolution of his symptoms later [5].

In contrast to the above reports, there are a few studies that failed to document any significant link between e-cigarette use and gastrointestinal disorders. In 2022, Debnath et al. investigated the effect of e-cigarettes on the gastrointestinal system by reviewing the data of the National Health and Nutrition Examination Survey (NHANES) between 2017 and 2018. The authors found no significant difference in the history of vomiting and diarrhea (over the last 30 days) between e-cigarette users and those who never used e-cigarettes (10.73% vs. 8.64%, $p = 0.320$). The study group consisted of 944 participants, 261 of whom used e-cigarettes at least 1 day and 683 never used e-cigarettes [6]. In 2023, Alturki et al. reported a weak association between the prevalence of GERD and use of e-cigarettes ($p = 0.788$). The study group consisted of 397 participants, 43.1% of whom were smokers, among whom one third (35%) were e-cigarette smokers [7]. Using a cross-sectional study on 273 e-cigarette users, Zein et al. reported the prevalence of GERD in only 5.5% of the cases. The authors used the GERD questionnaire with a cut-off score of 8. The most commonly reported reflux symptoms were regurgitation and heartburn in 10.3% and 6.6% of the cases, respectively. There was no significant association between duration or amount of e-cigarette use and heartburn, regurgitation, or nocturnal symptoms [8].

Why the high prevalence of GI symptoms in e-cigarette users? The high prevalence of GI symptoms in e-cigarette users is not surprising given the well-known impact of conventional smoking on the GI system. Numerous studies have shown that traditional smoking increases the risk of GI disorders. In a large meta-analysis on the risk factors for gastrointestinal symptoms, Eusebi et al. noted that smokers were at a higher risk than non-smokers with an odds ratio of 1.26. The prevalence of gastroesophageal reflux symptoms increased with obesity, the intake of non-steroidal anti-inflammatory drugs, and in patients above the age of 50 years [9]. In a review on the etiologic role of smoking in functional gastrointestinal disorders, Ohlsson noted that smokers had a 50% increased risk for functional dyspepsia [10]. Eastwood et al. reviewed the pathogenesis of peptic ulcer disease and found that smokers were more likely to develop ulcers and were less likely to heal than non-smokers [11].

Although there are no studies on the pathophysiology of GI disorders in e-cigarette users, there are many on the pathophysiology of GI symptoms in traditional cigarette smokers. The most commonly suggested mechanism is an increase in gastric acid secretion. Numerous studies showed that smoking and nicotine increase acid output by stimulating H2-receptors and enhancing the secretory function of parietal cells. Nicotine has also been shown to augment the secretion of pepsin, which has a detrimental effect on the mucosa, by increasing the number and secretory function of chief cells. This effect is compounded by the increase in gastric bile salt concentration and reflux of duodenal contents into the stomach, thus increasing the risk of gastric ulcer. Moreover, smoking has been associated with an increase in platelet-activating factor, a decrease in gastric mucosa prostaglandin secretion, and a decrease in gastric mucosa angiogenesis. All these factors act in concert to reduce the ability of the gastric mucosa to heal gastric ulcers [12]. Nicotine has also been shown to alter lower esophageal sphincter function, thus weakening its role as an anti-reflux barrier [13–15]. In a review on tobacco smoking and GERD, Ness-Jensen and Lagregren pointed out that tobacco smoking reduces lower esophageal sphincter pressure and hence facilitates reflux into the esophagus [16]. In an animal study, Tugay et al. noted impairment in gastric smooth muscle reactivity following exposure to acid reflux. There was an increased nicotine-induced relaxant response and a decrease in contractility of gastric smooth muscles, suggesting an etiologic role of nicotine in GERD [17]. Kahrilas and Gupta reported a decrease in lower esophageal sphincter pressure and an increase in the rate of acid reflux events in cigarette smokers compared to non-smokers. The majority of the events had occurred during deep inspiration or coughing [18]. These reports concur with a previous study by Rattan and Goyal, in which the authors showed that administration of nicotine sulfate intravenously resulted in a reduction in lower esophageal sphincter pressure. The dose-dependent effect was ascribed to the impact of nicotine on the noncholinergic and non-adrenergic inhibitory neurons [19]. With the decrease in lower esophageal sphincter pressure, there is an increased risk of reflux disease. Kadakia et al. conducted a study on the effect of cigarette smoking on gastroesophageal reflux disease and noted that cigarette smoking increased the percentage time during which the pH was less than 4 by 3.73%, and increased the number of reflux events [20]. To further support this hypothesis, Ness-Jensen et al. reported an association between smoking cessation, and improvement in GER symptoms with an adjusted IR of 1.78 in non-obese individuals using anti-reflux treatment at least weakly [21]. In conclusion, there is strong evidence in the literature to suggest that nicotine, which is a common ingredient in traditional and e-cigarettes, aggravates gastric aggressive behavior and weakens its defensive behavior.

Smoking may also predispose to reflux disease by altering salivary flow, pH, and its electrolyte concentration [22]. As noted in Chap. 8 on “Impact of E-Cigarette Smoking on Oral Cavity,” vaping often leads to changes in salivary flow and concentration. There is also growing evidence that smoking reduces the salivary concentration of epidermal growth factors [12]. Salivary growth factors play multiple roles in tissue repair and the maintenance of oral health. In addition to their role in adjusting salivary flow, salivary epidermal growth factors help promote oral mucosal healing by stimulating epithelial cell proliferation, migration, and differentiation [23]. Given the paramount role of saliva as a buffer to acidic reflux and its role in attenuating reflux symptoms, it is intuitive to conclude that the salivary changes due to smoking may exacerbate reflux-related symptoms and signs.

Laryngopharyngeal Reflux in E-Cigarette Users with Hoarseness

Laryngopharyngeal reflux (LPR) is a common inflammatory condition that affects 5–30% of the general population [24–27]. It is estimated that up to 30% of patients presenting to the otolaryngology clinic and more than 50% of those with voice disorders have LPR. In one study, which included 113 patients with dysphonia, Koufman et al. reported abnormal reflux testing in 73% of the cases [28]. Laryngopharyngeal reflux is characterized by retrograde movement of the gastroduodenal contents into the laryngopharynx. The term was initially coined in 1991 to describe atypical reflux in patients who present with symptoms related to the larynx and pharynx in the absence of heartburn and regurgitation [29]. Affected patients complain of a myriad of symptoms, including hoarseness, globus sensation, sticky mucus, post-nasal drip, and frequent throat clearing. Other symptoms such as dysphagia, odynophagia, cough, and ear pressure are also reported [30]. On laryngeal examination, there is hypertrophy of the posterior commissure, inflammatory changes in the mucosa overlying the arytenoids, and increased mucus [31–33].

There are no studies in the literature on the prevalence of LPR in e-cigarette users with or without hoarseness. However, as noted at the start of this chapter, there are many studies asserting that e-cigarette users experience esophageal and extraesophageal symptoms suggestive of reflux disease. Given that one out of three patients with GER disease has LPR symptoms and given the high prevalence of GER symptoms in e-cigarette users, one can extrapolate that e-cigarette users who experience symptoms of GER are more likely to have LPR [34, 35]. In one study, which included 167 patients with reflux esophagitis, Lai et al. noted the prevalence of LPR in almost one out of four participants [36]. Based on the above, reflux disease in e-cigarette users may be one of the risk factors for voice disorders.

Laryngopharyngeal reflux has been associated with structural and functional voice disorders [37–41]. In one study, Wang et al. showed a higher expression of pepsin in patients with vocal fold polyps compared to controls (75% vs. 31.25%; $P < 0.001$). The authors used 24-h impedance-pH monitoring and immunohistochemical analysis of tissue samples from polyps [42]. The pathogenesis of voice disorders in patients with LPR is complex and still under investigation. One of the reasons is the large disparity in laryngeal findings on endoscopy and the poor correlation between laryngeal signs and the frequency and severity of LPR symptoms. Several mechanisms have been suggested; one is the increase in mucus viscosity and dehydration. In addition to the decrease in bicarbonate secretion, acidic pepsin in the refluxate material has been shown to downregulate mucin genes and reduce the production of MUC4 and MUC5AC expression [43, 44]. Mucins play a vital role in hydrating and lubricating the vocal folds. The increased viscosity of the mucus overlying the vocal fold cover has a negative effect on vocal fold vibration, resulting in an increase in aperiodicity and a decrease in amplitude [45]. Another suggested mechanism is vocal fold cell dehiscence and trauma. There is strong evidence suggesting that exposure of the laryngeal mucosa to the refluxate material disrupts the epithelial junctional complexes and hence the epithelial barrier. Studies have shown the presence of pepsin in the laryngeal epithelium, both intra- and extracellular [46–49]. When activated at a pH between 1.5 and 6, pepsin can cause cellular injury, such as mitochondrial damage [50–52]. Pepsin also plays a role in the recruitment of inflammatory cells and angiogenesis, which may explain the signs of inflammation on laryngeal examination. There is also a decrease in e-cadherin expression and dilatation of the intracellular vocal epithelium space [44, 53, 54]. The Reinke's space is also affected by laryngopharyngeal reflux. Pepsin plays a role in regulating the water volume across the vocal fold cover. Dehydration of the superficial layer of the lamina propria also affects the pliability of the vocal fold cover. Last but not least, hoarseness in patients with LPR can be secondary to laryngeal hyperfunction as a compensatory behavior to the decrease in voice efficiency.

References

1. Li Q, Zhan Y, Wang L, Leischow SJ, Zeng DD. Analysis of symptoms and their potential associations with e-liquids' components: a social media study. BMC Public Health. 2016;16:1–2.
2. Farooqi W, Hussamuldin A, Alabdullah A, Albatati A, Alshathri FS, Alabdullah S, Alzuhair A. Prevalence of gastroesophageal reflux disease (GERD) among electronic cigarette-smoking university students in Riyadh, Saudi Arabia. Cureus. 2024;16(12)
3. Camus M, Gallois G, Marteau P. Ulcerative colitis and electronic cigarette: what's the matter? Am Coll Gastroenteroll ACG. 2014;109(4):608–9.
4. Pasricha TS, Kochar B. Vaping-associated esophagitis. BMC Gastroenterol. 2021;21:1–3.
5. Pace LM, McGoogan K. Vaping induced severe erosive esophagitis. JPGN Rep. 2023;4(3):e327.
6. Debnath M, Debnath D, Singh P, Wert Y, Nookala V. Effect of electronic cigarettes on the gastrointestinal system. Cureus. 2022;14(7)
7. Alturki NA, Alghamdi RA, Almehmadi RG, Derar RM, Waznah RM, Niyazi RA, Hasrat GS, Alfayez FF, Elsamanoudy A, Derar RM II, Waznah R. Prevalence of gastroesophageal reflux disease (GERD) among electronic cigarette-smoking university students in Jeddah, Saudi Arabia. Cureus. 2023;15(3)
8. Zein AF, Nauphar D, Khasanah U, Pratamawati TM, Brajawikalpa RS, Ayuningtyas E, Hamzah A. The association between the pattern of electronic cigarette smoking and gastroesophageal reflux. Indones J Gastroenterol Hepatol Dig Endosc. 2021;22(1):16–20.
9. Eusebi LH, Ratnakumaran R, Yuan Y, Solaymani-Dodaran M, Bazzoli F, Ford AC. Global prevalence of, and risk factors for, gastro-oesophageal reflux symptoms: a meta-analysis. Gut. 2018;67(3):430–40. https://doi.org/10.1136/gutjnl-2016-313589. Epub 2017 Feb 23. PMID: 28232473.
10. Ohlsson B. The role of smoking and alcohol behaviour in management of functional gastrointestinal disorders. Best Pract Res Clin Gastroenterol. 2017;31(5):545–52.
11. Eastwood GL. Is smoking still important in the pathogenesis of peptic ulcer disease? J Clin Gastroenterol. 1997;25:S1–7.
12. Maity P, Biswas K, Roy S, Banerjee RK, Bandyopadhyay U. Smoking and the pathogenesis of gastroduodenal ulcer—recent mechanistic update. Mol Cell Biochem. 2003;253(1–2):329–38. https://doi.org/10.1023/a:1026040723669. PMID: 14619984.
13. Miller LS, Vegesna AK, Braverman AS, Barbe MF, Ruggieri MR Sr. Enhanced nicotinic receptor mediated relaxations in gastroesophageal muscle fibers from Barrett's esophagus patients. Neurogastroenterol Motil. 2014;26(3):430–9. https://doi.org/10.1111/nmo.12294. Epub 2013 Dec 15. PMID: 24330081; PMCID: PMC4019224.
14. Wang F, Li G, Ning J, Chen L, Xu H, Kong X, Bu J, Zhao W, Li Z, Wang X, Li X, Ma J. Alcohol accumulation promotes esophagitis via pyroptosis activation. Int J Biol Sci.

2018;14(10):1245–55. https://doi.org/10.7150/ijbs.24347. PMID: 30123073; PMCID: PMC6097477.

15. Rom O, Pecorelli A, Valacchi G, Reznick AZ. Are e-cigarettes a safe and good alternative to cigarette smoking? Ann N Y Acad Sci. 2015;1340:65–74. https://doi.org/10.1111/nyas.12609. Epub 2014 Dec 31. PMID: 25557889.
16. Ness-Jensen E, Lagergren J. Tobacco smoking, alcohol consumption and gastro-oesophageal reflux disease. Best Pract Res Clin Gastroenterol. 2017;31(5):501–8.
17. Tugay M, Yildiz F, Utkan Z, Utkan T, Sarioğlu Y. Impaired gastric motility in the gastroesophageal reflux rat model: an in vitro study. J Surg Res. 2003;115(2):272–8.
18. Kahrilas PJ, Gupta RR. Mechanisms of acid reflux associated with cigarette smoking. Gut. 1990;31(1):4–10.
19. Rattan S, Goyal RK. Effect of nicotine on the lower esophageal sphincter: studies on the mechanism of action. Gastroenterology. 1975;69(1):154–9.
20. Kadakia SC, Kikendall JW, Maydonovitch C, Johnson LF. Effect of cigarette smoking on gastroesophageal reflux measured by 24-h ambulatory esophageal pH monitoring. Am J Gastroenterol. 1995;90(10).
21. Ness-Jensen E, Lindam A, Lagergren J, Hveem K. Tobacco smoking cessation and improved gastroesophageal reflux: a prospective population-based cohort study: the HUNT study. Am Coll GastroenterolIACG. 2014;109:171.
22. Zięba S, Zalewska A, Żukowski P, Maciejczyk M. Can smoking alter salivary homeostasis? A systematic review on the effects of traditional and electronic cigarettes on qualitative and quantitative saliva parameters. Dent Med Probl. 2024;61(1):129–44.
23. Royce LS, Baum BJ. Physiologic levels of salivary epidermal growth factor stimulate migration of an oral epithelial cell line. Biochim Biophys Acta. 1991;1092(3):401–3. https://doi.org/10.1016/s0167-4889(97)90019-7. PMID: 2049404.
24. Li J, Zhang L, Zhang C, Cheng JY, Li J, Jeff Cheng CF. Linguistic adaptation, reliability, validation, and responsivity of the Chinese version of Reflux Symptom Index. J Voice. 2016;30:104–8.
25. Chen XM, Li Y, Guo WL, Wang WT, Lu M. Prevalence of laryngopharyngeal reflux disease in Fuzhou region of China. Zhonghua Er Bi Yan Hou Tou Jing Wai Ke Za Zhi. 2016;51:909–13.
26. Spantideas N, Drosou E, Bougea A, Assimakopoulos D. Laryngopharyngeal reflux disease in the Greek general population, prevalence and risk factors. BMC Ear Nose Throat Disord. 2015;15:7.
27. Kamani T, Penney S, Mitra I, Pothula V. The prevalence of laryngopharyngeal reflux in the English population. Eur Arch Otorrinolaringol. 2012;269:2219–25.
28. Koufman JA, Amin MR, Panetti M. Prevalence of reflux in 113 consecutive patients with laryngeal and voice disorders. Otolaryngol Head Neck Surg. 2000;123:385–8.
29. Koufman JA. The otolaryngologic manifestations of gastroesophageal reflux disease (GERD): a clinical investigation of 225 patients using ambulatory 24-hour pH monitoring and an experimental investigation of the role of acid and pepsin in the development of laryngeal injury. Laryngoscope. 1991;101(4 pt 2 suppl 53):1–78.
30. Ren JJ, Zhao Y, Wang J, et al. PepsinA as a marker of laryngopharyngeal reflux detected in chronic rhinosinusitis patients. Otolaryngol Head Neck Surg. 2017;156:893–900.
31. Habermann W, Schmid C, Neumann K, et al. Reflux Symptom Index and Reflux Finding Score in otolaryngologic practice. J Voice. 2012;26:e123–7.
32. Lee YS, Choi SH, Son YI, Park YH, Kim SY, Nam SY. Prospective, observational study using rabeprazole in 455 patients with laryngopharyngeal reflux disease. Eur Arch Otorrinolaringol. 2011;268:863–9.
33. Chappity P, Kumar R, Deka RC, Chokkalingam V, Saraya A, Sikka K. Proton pump inhibitors versus solitary lifestyle modification in management of laryngopharyngeal reflux and evaluating who is at risk: scenario in a developing country. Clin Med Insights Ear Nose Throat. 2014;7:1–5.

34. Groome M, Cotton JP, Borland M, McLeod S, Johnston DA, Dillon JF. Prevalence of laryngopharyngeal reflux in a population with gastroesophageal reflux. Laryngoscope. 2007;117:1424–8.
35. Jaspersen D, Kulig M, Labenz J, et al. Prevalence of extra-oesophageal manifestations in gastro-oesophageal reflux disease: an analysis based on the ProGERD study. Aliment Pharmacol Ther. 2003;17:1515–20.
36. Lai Y-C, Wang P, Lin J. Laryngopharyngeal reflux in patients with reflux esophagitis. World J Gastroenterol. 2008;14(28):4523.
37. Ward PH, Zwitman D, Hanson D, Berci G. Contact ulcers and granulomas of the larynx: new insights into their etiology as a basis for more rational treatment. Otolaryngol Head Neck Surg (1979). 1980;88(3):262–9.
38. Koufman JA, Wiener GJ, Wu WC, Castell DO. Reflux laryngitis and its sequelae: the diagnostic role of ambulatory 24-hour pH monitoring. J Voice. 1988;2(1):78–89.
39. Ross JA, Noordzji JP, Woo P. Voice disorders in patients with suspected laryngo-pharyngeal reflux disease. J Voice. 1998;12(1):84–8.
40. Rothstein SG. Reflux and vocal disorders in singers with bulimia. J Voice. 1998;12(1):89–90.
41. Kuhn J, Toohill RJ, Ulualp SO, Kulpa J, Hofmann C, Arndorfer R, Shaker R. Pharyngeal acid reflux events in patients with vocal cord nodules. Laryngoscope. 1998;108(8 Pt 1):1146–9.
42. Wang L, Tan JJ, Wu T, Zhang R, Wu JN, Zeng FF, Liu YL, Han XY, Li YF, Li XP. Association between laryngeal pepsin levels and the presence of vocal fold polyps. Otolaryngol Head Neck Surg. 2017;156(1):144–51.
43. Voynow JA, Gendler SJ, Rose MC. Regulation of mucin genes in chronic inflammatory airway diseases. Am J Respir Cell Mol Biol. 2006;34:661–5.
44. Johnston N, Bulmer D, Gill GA, et al. Cell biology of laryngeal epithelial defenses in health and disease: further studies. Ann Otol Rhinol Laryngol. 2003;112:481–91.
45. Nakagawa H, Fukuda H, Kawaida M, et al. Lubrication mechanism of the larynx during phonation: an experiment in excised canine larynges. Folia Phoniatr Logop. 1998;50:183–94.
46. Bulmer DM, Ali MS, Brownlee IA, et al. Laryngeal mucosa: its susceptibility to damage by acid and pepsin. Laryngoscope. 2010;120:777–82.
47. Jiang A, Liang M, Su Z, et al. Immunohistochemical detection of pepsin in laryngeal mucosa for diagnosing laryngopharyngeal reflux. Laryngoscope. 2011;121:1426–30.
48. Durkes A, Sivasankar MP. Bicarbonate availability for vocal fold epithelial defense to acidic challenge. Ann Otol Rhinol Laryngol. 2014;123:71–6.
49. Na SY, Kwon OE, Lee YC, et al. Optimal timing of saliva collection to detect pepsin in patients with laryngopharyngeal reflux. Laryngoscope. 2016;126:2770–3.
50. Ylitalo R, Thibeault SL. Relationship between time of exposure of laryngopharyngeal reflux and gene expression in laryngeal fibroblasts. Ann Otol Rhinol Laryngol. 2006;115:775–83.
51. Johnston N, Dettmar PW, Bishwokarma B, et al. Activity/stability of human pepsin: implications for reflux attributed laryngeal disease. Laryngoscope. 2007;117:1036–9.
52. Johnston N, Wells CW, Samuels TL, et al. Pepsin in nonacidic refluxate can damage hypopharyngeal epithelial cells. Ann Otol Rhinol Laryngol. 2009;118:677–85.
53. Gill GA, Johnston N, Buda A, et al. Laryngeal epithelial defenses against laryngopharyngeal reflux: investigations of E-cadherin, carbonic anhydrase isoenzyme III, and pepsin. Ann Otol Rhinol Laryngol. 2005;114:913–21.
54. Reichel O, Mayr D, Durst F, et al. E-cadherin but not beta-catenin expression is decreased in laryngeal biopsies from patients with laryngopharyngeal reflux. Eur Arch Otorrinolaringol. 2008;265:937–42.

Impact of E-Cigarettes on the Neurologic System 11

The impact of e-cigarettes on various systems in the body has been described in numerous animal studies and clinical trials. The adverse neurologic events in particular have gained special attention in view of the significant use of e-cigarettes among youngsters and adolescents [1–3]. Seiler-Ramadas et al. reported headache, irritability, anxiety, depression, and insomnia as common neurologic complaints in e-cigarette smokers in addition to clusters of other symptoms related to different organs [4]. Hua et al. extracted data on the health effects of e-cigarette smoking from online forum posts of 41,216 vapers and noted the neurological system as the most severely affected system in the body. Described complaints included headache, malaise, dizziness, fatigue, and migraine [5]. King et al. examined the prevalence of six symptoms thought to be caused by e-cigarettes using a nationally representative cross-sectional survey of US youth that included 975 participants between the ages of 13 and 17 years. Their results showed that dizziness and headache were the second and third most frequently reported symptoms in 31.5% and 25.4% of the cases, respectively. The authors stressed the need to educate healthcare providers about the nature of these health symptoms and their correlation with vaping [6]. E-cigarettes have also been implicated in the exacerbation of new-onset seizures [7–9]. Faulcon et al. reported 122 cases of seizures, 7 cases of syncope, and one case of tremor associated with the use of electronic nicotine delivery systems. Eighty-five percent of those who reported seizures noted their occurrence within 24 h of last use [10]. Talum and Oster described two cases of new-onset seizures that occurred within hours of vaping. The cases were identified using a survey sent to 30 healthcare-related staff who were asked if they had inquired about the use of e-cigarettes in patients presenting with new-onset seizures. One patient used a cannabinoid-based product while the other used a nicotine-based product [11].

Animal studies have also shown that e-cigarette smoking may lead to memory impairment. Alzoubi et al. conducted an animal study looking at the effects of e-cigarette aerosol on learning and memory function in Wistar rats. Following a whole-body exposure to the aerosol, 1 h a day for 4 and 12 weeks, the authors

A.-l. Hamdan, *E-Cigarette Smoking, Voice, and Health*,
https://doi.org/10.1007/978-3-032-04913-1_11

reported a decrease in the activity of anti-oxidant enzymes in the hippocampus and a reduction in short-and long-term memory [12]. Using mice that were fed a high-fat diet for 16 weeks and exposed to tobacco-flavored e-vapor with and without nicotine, Chen et al. reported a significant impairment in short-term memory function 15 weeks later. The impairment in short-term memory was independent of the nicotine and or diet, and was associated with an increase in systemic inflammation [13].

Pathophysiology of Adverse Effects of Vaping on the Neurologic System

The adverse effects of vaping on the neurologic system can be attributed to the impact of the chemical compounds in e-cigarettes, including nicotine [14]. In an animal study on brain nicotine kinetics, Sai et al. reported a rapid surge and sharp increase in the nicotine concentration in the brain following a single puff [15]. Numerous studies on conventional cigarettes showed that nicotine may induce neurologic deficits such as addiction, cognitive dysfunction, stroke, neuroinflammation, and neurogenic developmental dysfunction [16]. Nicotine plays a central role in the neural system via the nicotine acetylcholine receptors (nAChRs), which are pentameric ion channels widely distributed in various neuroanatomical areas. Henderson et al. investigated the impact of vaporized nicotine on neuronal function in an animal model using mice that were exposed to a 20-session e-Vape self-administration and noted changes in neuronal excitability following exposure [17]. Nicotine also has a substantial impact on the limbic-dopaminergic system, which plays a crucial role in regulating reward-driven behaviors and emotions, particularly in adolescents [18–20]. The adolescent brain undergoes various alterations associated with an increase in functional connectivity and substantial neurochemical maturation that involves particularly the dopaminergic system [21–25]. Numerous studies have shown that chronic exposure to nicotine in adolescents can alter the brain neurochemistry, resulting in neurobiological sensitization and changes in neuronal signaling [26]. In addition to its impact on dopamine regulation, it also alters indices of serotonin receptors with a long-lasting detrimental effect on serotonergic signaling [27–29].

Based on the above, many of the adverse neurologic events associated with vaping can be ascribed, at least partially, to the nicotine content in e-cigarette aerosol. This is in accord with studies further documenting dysfunction in the brain lipid profile of e-cigarette users. Cardenia et al. investigated the effect of electronic-cigarette aerosol on rat brain lipid profile using two male Sprague Dawley rats that were exposed to 11 cycles per day for 5 days a week for a total of 8 weeks. The results indicated that e-cigarette aerosol disturbed the lipid and cholesterol homeostasis, which could increase the risk of neurodegenerative diseases. For instance, there was a decrease in cholesterol at 8 weeks in those exposed to the aerosol in comparison to controls (21.57 mg/g vs. 24.56 mg/g, respectively) [30]. The neuropathophysiologic changes associated with e-cigarette use can also be attributed to the non-nicotinic chemical compounds present in e-cigarettes. E-cigarette non-nicotinic constituents also have an impact on the central nervous system regulatory component, such as the blood–brain barrier. Heldt investigated the impact of e-cigarette use on blood–brain barrier function using sequencing of microvessel RNA. The results showed a decrease in the expression of Occludin and Glut 1, and a downregulation of many genes that play a crucial role in BBB function. The authors also noted a decrease in novel object recognition in mice following exposure to nicotine-free e-cigarettes. The authors stressed the adverse effect of e-cigarettes on the neurovascular system [31]. E-cigarette use also has an effect on the rat brain lipid profile in animal studies.

References

1. Esteban-Lopez M, Perry MD, Garbinski LD, et al. Health effects and known pathology associated with the use of e-cigarettes. Toxicol Rep. 2022;9:1357–68. https://doi.org/10.1016/j.toxrep.2022.06.006. PMID: 36561957; PMCID: PMC9764206.
2. Lieu TA, Bibbins-Domingo K. E-cigarette use in adolescents and adults—a JAMA collection. JAMA. 2024;332(9):709–10.
3. Battista K, Patte KA, Wade TJ, Cole AG, Elton-Marshall T, Lucibello KM, Pickett W, Leatherdale ST. Do sociodemographic risk profiles for adolescents engaging in weekly e-cigarette, cigarette, and dual product use differ? BMC Public Health. 2024;24(1):1558.
4. Seiler-Ramadas R, Sandner I, Haider S, Grabovac I, Dorner TE. Health effects of electronic cigarette (e-cigarette) use on organ systems and its implications for public health. Wien Klin Wochenschr. 2021;133(19–20):1020–7. https://doi.org/10.1007/s00508-020-01711-z. Epub 2020 Jul 20. PMID: 32691214; PMCID: PMC8500897.
5. Hua M, Sadah S, Hristidis V, Talbot P. Health effects associated with electronic cigarette use: automated mining of online forums. J Med Internet Res. 2020;22(1):e15684. https://doi.org/10.2196/15684. PMID: 31899452; PMCID: PMC6969389.
6. King JL, Reboussin BA, Merten JW, Wiseman KD, Wagoner KG, Sutfin EL. Negative health symptoms reported by youth e-cigarette users: results from a national survey of US youth. Addict Behav. 2020;104:106315. https://doi.org/10.1016/j.addbeh.2020.106315. Epub 2020 Jan 13. PMID: 31981796; PMCID: PMC8055041.
7. Michael Felberbaum. FDA In Brief: FDA encourages continued submission of reports related to seizures following e-cigarette use as part of agency's ongoing scientific investigation of potential safety issue2019. https://www.fda.gov/news-events/fda-brief/fda-brief-fda-encourages-continued-submission-reports-related-seizures-following-e-cigarette-use. Accessed 4 Feb 2021.
8. Quezada T, Sianati B, Valeriano J. Vaping and seizure risk: a case report (1814). Neurology. 2020;94(15_supplement):1814.
9. Oster J, Tatum P, Monigan C, Kryzanski J. E-cigarette use (vaping) causes seizures on EEG detected by responsive neurstimulation: evidence from electrocorticography (1809). Neurology. 2020;94(15_supplement):1809.
10. Faulcon LM, Rudy S, Limpert J, Wang B, Murphy I. Adverse experience reports of seizures in youth and young adult electronic nicotine delivery systems users. J Adolesc Health. 2020;66(1):15–7. https://doi.org/10.1016/j.jadohealth.2019.10.002. PMID: 31866055.
11. Tatum PS, Oster JM. Seizures and vaping—a report of two cases. Mil Med. 2023;188(5–6):e1307–9. https://doi.org/10.1093/milmed/usab270. PMID: 34272954.
12. Alzoubi KH, Batran RM, Al-Sawalha NA, Khabour OF, Karaoghlanian N, Shihadeh A, Eissenberg T. The effect of electronic cigarettes exposure on learning and memory functions:

behavioral and molecular analysis. Inhal Toxicol. 2021;33(6–8):234–43. https://doi.org/10.1080/08958378.2021.1954732. Epub 2021 Jul 27. PMID: 34311661; PMCID: PMC9270881.
13. Chen H, Wang B, Li G, Steele JR, Stayte S, Vissel B, Chan YL, Yi C, Saad S, Machaalani R, Oliver BG. Brain health is independently impaired by e-vaping and high-fat diet. Brain Behav Immun. 2021;92:57–66. https://doi.org/10.1016/j.bbi.2020.11.028. Epub 2020 Nov 20. PMID: 33221488.
14. Staal YCM, Li Y, Gerber LS, Fokkens P, Cremers H, Cassee FR, Talhout R, Westerink RHS, Heusinkveld HJ. Neuromodulatory and neurotoxic effects of e-cigarette vapor using a realistic exposure method. Inhal Toxicol. 2023;35(3–4):76–85. https://doi.org/10.1080/08958378.2022.2118911. Epub 2022 Sep 2. PMID: 36053669.
15. Solingapuram Sai KK, Zuo Y, Rose JE, Garg PK, Garg S, Nazih R, Mintz A, Mukhin AG. Rapid brain nicotine uptake from electronic cigarettes. J Nucl Med. 2020;61(6):928–30. https://doi.org/10.2967/jnumed.119.230748. Epub 2019 Nov 1. PMID: 31676729; PMCID: PMC8008769.
16. López-Ojeda W, Hurley RA. Vaping and the brain: effects of electronic cigarettes and e-liquid substances. J Neuropsychiatry Clin Neurosci. 2024;36(1):A41–5. https://doi.org/10.1176/appi.neuropsych.20230184. PMID: 38226910.
17. Henderson BJ, Young LE, Olszewski NA, Tetteh-Quarshie S, Maddox SK, Simpkins MA, Dudich MC, McGlauglin MS, Weinsweig ZC, Cooper SY. Age-dependent effects of vaping on the prefrontal cortex, ventral tegmental area, and nucleus accumbens. Commun Biol. 2024;7(1):1553. https://doi.org/10.1038/s42003-024-07272-5. PMID: 39572675; PMCID: PMC11582578.
18. Yuan M, Cross SJ, Loughlin SE, Leslie FM. Nicotine and the adolescent brain. J Physiol. 2015;593(16) https://doi.org/10.1113/jp270492.
19. Xia W, Veljkovic E, Koshibu K, Peitsch MC, Hoeng J. Neurobehavioral effects of selected tobacco constituents in rodents following subchronic administration. Eur J Pharmacol. 2019;865:865. https://doi.org/10.1016/j.ejphar.2019.172809.
20. John U, Meyer C, Rumpf HJ, Hapke U. Smoking, nicotine dependence and psychiatric comorbidity—a population-based study including smoking cessation after three years. Drug Alcohol Depend. 2004;76:287–95. https://doi.org/10.1016/j.drugalcdep.2004.06.004.
21. Hwang K, Velanova K, Luna B. Strengthening of top-down frontal cognitive control networks underlying the development of inhibitory control: a functional magnetic resonance imaging effective connectivity study. J Neurosci. 2010;30:15535–45. https://doi.org/10.1523/JNEUROSCI.2825-10.2010.
22. Fair DA, Cohen AL, Power JD, Dosenbach NU, Church JA, Miezin FM, Schlaggar BL, Petersen SE. Functional brain networks develop from a "local to distributed" organization. PLoS Comput Biol. 2009;5:e1000381. https://doi.org/10.1371/journal.pcbi.1000381.
23. Teicher MH, Andersen SL, Hostetter JC. Evidence for dopamine receptor pruning between adolescence and adulthood in striatum but not nucleus accumbens. Dev Brain Res. 1995;89:167–72. https://doi.org/10.1016/0165-3806(95)00109-q.
24. Brenhouse HC, Sonntag KC, Andersen SL. Transient D1 dopamine receptor expression on prefrontal cortex projection neurons: relationship to enhanced motivational salience of drug cues in adolescence. J Neurosci. 2008;28:2375–82. https://doi.org/10.1523/JNEUROSCI.5064-07.2008.
25. Naneix F, Marchand AR, Di Scala G, Pape JR, Coutureau E. Parallel maturation of goal-directed behavior and dopaminergic systems during adolescence. J Neurosci. 2012;32:16223–32. https://doi.org/10.1523/JNEUROSCI.3080-12.2012.
26. McQuown SC, Dao JM, Belluzzi JD, Leslie FM. Age-dependent effects of low-dose nicotine treatment on cocaine-induced behavioral plasticity in rats. Psychopharmacology. 2009;207:143–52. https://doi.org/10.1007/s00213-009-1642-0.
27. Xu Z, Seidler FJ, Cousins MM, Slikker W Jr, Slotkin TA. Adolescent nicotine administration alters serotonin receptors and cell signaling mediated through adenylyl cyclase. Brain Res. 2002;951:280–92. https://doi.org/10.1016/s0006-8993(02)03174-8.

28. Slotkin TA, Card J, Seidler FJ. Nicotine administration in adolescence reprograms the subsequent response to nicotine treatment and withdrawal in adulthood: sex-selective effects on cerebrocortical serotonergic function. Brain Res Bull. 2014;102:1–8. https://doi.org/10.1016/j.brainresbull.2014.01.004.
29. Slotkin TA, Seidler FJ. Nicotine exposure in adolescence alters the response of serotonin systems to nicotine administered subsequently in adulthood. Dev Neurosci. 2009;31:58–70. https://doi.org/10.1159/000207494.
30. Cardenia V, Vivarelli F, Cirillo S, Paolini M, Canistro D, Rodriguez-Estrada MT. The effect of electronic-cigarettes aerosol on rat brain lipid profile. Biochimie. 2018;153:99–108. https://doi.org/10.1016/j.biochi.2018.07.027. Epub 2018 Aug 2. PMID: 30077815.
31. Heldt NA, Seliga A, Winfield M, Gajghate S, Reichenbach N, Yu X, Rom S, Tenneti A, May D, Gregory BD, Persidsky Y. Electronic cigarette exposure disrupts blood-brain barrier integrity and promotes neuroinflammation. Brain Behav Immun. 2020;88:363–80. https://doi.org/10.1016/j.bbi.2020.03.034. Epub 2020 Mar 31. PMID: 32243899; PMCID: PMC7899242.

Risk of Cancer in E-Cigarette Users

12

The surge in the popularity of e-cigarettes has instigated ongoing research on their safety despite being advertised as a safe alternative to conventional cigarettes. In addition to their adverse effects on various systems in the body, their potential oncogenicity is a growing concern among healthcare providers. An increasing number of scientific reports are providing new lines of evidence suggesting that vaping increases the risk of cancer, although a cause-and-effect relation remains elusive. This ambiguity of conception on the link between vaping and cancer is partly due to the lag period between exposure and oncogenic transformation. The expansion of e-cigarette use in the last decade precludes having enough epidemiological evidence on the long-term effects of vaping. A second reason is that a large percentage of vapers are dual smokers, which masks the isolated oncogenic effect of e-cigarettes. One must also note that most in vitro studies published were conducted on cell lines exposed to e-cigarette aerosol in a laboratory setting that is remotely distinct from real human exposure. Future research imitating in vivo conditions of vaping is needed to establish unequivocal evidence that e-cigarettes are carcinogenic [1–3].

Nevertheless, there is ubiquity of reports showing that e-cigarette smoking induces biological and toxic alterations that increase the risk of cancer. Based on numerous studies, many of the chemical compounds of e-cigarettes are hazardous and cause cell damage, more so following the heating process [4]. Many investigators have shown that e-cigarette exposure can lead to changes in metabolic activity, cytotoxicity, apoptosis, DNA damage, meta-nuclear anomalies, oxidative stress, and an increase in inflammatory biomarkers [3, 5–16]. The extent of harm varies with the type of e-cigarette used, duration of exposure to e-cigarette vapors, and patterns of smoking. The cellular damage has been attributed mostly to the cytotoxicity of several ingredients of the e-cigarette liquid and aerosol, among which is nicotine. It is estimated that nicotine-based e-cigarettes contain between 3 mg and 36 mg of nicotine per milliliter and that 10% of inhaled nicotine is transformed into nitrosamine compounds [17, 18]. Nitrosamines are known for their carcinogenic potential by increasing DNA methylation [18]. DNA damage may also occur from

A.-l. Hamdan, *E-Cigarette Smoking, Voice, and Health*,
https://doi.org/10.1007/978-3-032-04913-1_12

exposure to other genotoxic compounds that could be primary or daughter products of vaping. These include carbonyl compounds such as formaldehyde, acetaldehyde, and acrolein [19–22]. Propylene glycol and glycerol, the main constituents of e-cigarette liquids commonly used to carry flavorings, are known to release formaldehyde during the evaporation process, which increases the risk of cancer according to many authors [22, 23]. Another carbonyl compound present in e-cigarette aerosol that has carcinogenic potential is acetaldehyde. Even at low dosage, acetaldehyde has been shown to induce DNA adducts and alter DNA replication, thus promoting cancerization of tissues [24, 25]. Acrolein, a chemical compound present in e-cigarette aerosol, has also been incriminated in the development of cancer in animal studies. Acrolein, a known toxic chemical present in e-cigarette aerosol, can induce TP53 mutational hotspots and the formation of DNA adducts [22]. Other hazardous compounds linked to e-cigarette smoking include menthol and ethyl maltol. Ethyl maltol, commonly present in flavored e-liquids to impart sweetness, has been associated with free radical generation once vaped, in addition to its inflammatory effect and ability to compromise local immune function. Bitzer et al. noted that ethyl maltol's enhanced free radical formation varied with the concentration used. Free radicals, in turn, have been linked to oncogenicity, which suggests that ethyl maltol may also carry an oncogenic potential [26–28]. Another toxic substance that is commonly added to e-cigarette liquid is vitamin E acetate. Thermal decomposition of this latter results in the release of toxic chemicals such as benzene and alkene, which in turn have potential carcinogenic activity [29]. Other compounds present in e-cigarettes that can be toxic and carcinogenic include metals such as chromium and nickel [29, 30]. Heavy-metal toxicity and oncogenicity have been linked to free-radical generation and reactive oxygen species.

Oral Cancer

Oral cancer is one of the most common cancers, ranking as the 18th most common malignancy in the world with hundreds of thousands of new cases diagnosed yearly [31]. Given its significant morbidity and high mortality rate, oral cancer represents a major public health and a challenge to the health care providers [32]. The most common type is squamous cell carcinoma, accounting for 90% of the cases, with the most significant risk factor being smoking [33–36]. Smoking can affect cell viability, causing DNA damage and promoting apoptotic cell signaling through nuclear receptors, thus increasing the risk of malignancy [37–40].

The last two decades witnessed the introduction of a new form of smoking that is less harmful than conventional cigarettes, namely e-cigarettes [41–43]. Since its inception, many adverse effects related to various organs and structures in the body have been described, including the oral cavity. The current literature indicates that e-cigarette smoking can lead to inflammatory diseases of the mucosa of the oral cavity, such as angular cheilitis and stomatitis [44, 45]. However, the oncogenicity of vaping in regard to the oral cavity remains inconclusive. What is well established is that exposure to e-cigarette aerosol has adverse effects on cell viability, leading to alterations in metabolic activity, an increase in apoptosis, oxidative stress, an increase in LDH enzyme, and DNA damage (DNA strand breaking and upregulation of TP53) [7, 8]. In 2016, Yu et al. showed that normal epithelial cells and head and neck squamous cell carcinoma cell lines had a reduction in cell viability following exposure to e-cigarette vapor with and without nicotine for 2–56 days. The authors stressed that e-cigarette vapor is cytotoxic and induces DNA damage [7]. The same year, Sancilio et al. exposed human gingival fibroblasts (HGF) to e-cigarette liquid with and without nicotine and showed an increase in reactive oxygen species (ROS) production after 24 h, and an increase in Bax expression, which plays a role in apoptosis, after 48 h [8]. Korrapati et al. investigated the cytotoxicity of e-cigarette vapor of various concentrations (0.5%, 1.0%, and 2.0% by volume) and noted a five-fold increase in epithelial cell death following short-term exposure. The rate of cell death increased when e-cigarette vapor with nicotine was used. The authors also found an increase in migration of head and neck squamous cell carcinoma cancer cells. In conclusion, they stressed the short-term carcinogenic effects of vaping [46]. In 2020, Vermehren et al. investigated the impact of e-cigarette vapor on HGF and noted a significantly higher metabolic activity after 1 h, 24 h, and 48 h. There was no significant difference in the extent of apoptosis between the HGF exposed to e-cigarette vapor vs. those exposed to cigarette smoke [6]. In 2023, Muniz de Lima demonstrated in an in vitro study that e-liquid can promote proliferation and invasion of normal and abnormal oral epithelial cells [9].

Many of these in vitro studies were substantiated by clinical reports. In 2018. Bustamante et al. conducted an analytical cross-sectional study in three groups of participants (e-cigarette smokers, smokers, and non-smokers) and noted the formation of *N*′-nitrosonornicotine (NNN) in the saliva of e-cigarette users. The authors stressed the need to consider e-cigarette smoking as a health risk factor given that NNN is a tobacco-specific oral carcinogen [47]. In 2019, Tommasi et al. investigated gene regulation in oral cells of e-cigarette users and noted dysregulation of key genes with convergence toward cancer-related pathways in many. The authors used oral cells that were submitted to transcriptome analysis [48]. In 2020, Ye et al. conducted a cross-sectional study looking at the impact of e-cigarettes on biologic profiles of saliva and gingival crevicular fluid derived from volunteer participants who were divided into four groups: conventional smoking, e-cigarette smokers, dual smokers, and non-smokers. There was a statistically significant difference in biomarkers of inflammatory mediators between dual smokers and e-cigarette users. The authors also found statistically significant differences in myeloperoxidase and matrix metalloproteinase-9 between e-cigarette users and non-smokers [15]. In 2021, using saliva of smokers, non-smokers, and vapors, Pandarathodiyil et al. showed that e-vapor exposure resulted in an increase in LDH levels in comparison to controls, with no significant difference in comparison to conventional smokers. The authors alluded to the cytotoxic effect of e-cigarettes on the oral mucosa [12]. That same year, Schwarzmeir et al. investigated the cytotoxicity and cytogenetic damage to the oral mucosa of e-cigarette users. The samples examined were smears of exfoliative cells taken from the lateral region of the tongue and floor of the mouth [11]. The results showed an increase in micronuclei frequency between smokers and controls. There were also significant differences in metanuclear anomalies, namely karyolysis, karyorrhexis, broken eggs, and nuclear bud, between e-cigarette users and controls. However, it is important to note that e-cigarette users in that study had a history of conventional cigarette smoking and alcohol consumption [11]. In 2022, Cheng et al. examined oral brushing and urine of 20 e-cigarette users and 8 smokers and noted higher levels of DNA adduct of acrolein in vapors compared to non-smokers [49]. In 2022, Kamal et al. reported an increase in inflammatory and cancer risk biomarkers in the saliva of e-cigarette users compared to non-smokers. There was an increase in salivary IL-1β and transforming growth factor-β following exposure to e-cigarette vapor, thus further substantiating the harm of e-cigarettes and associated increased risk for systemic diseases [50].

There were also four case reports in the literature implicating vaping as a risk factor for the development of oral cavity cancer. In 2014, Bartram et al. reported a 55-year-old case of florid oral lichen planus that was ascribed to e-cigarette smoking. The patient had presented with a white lesion on the buccal and upper and lower labial mucosa, and on the lateral border of the tongue. Microscopic examination revealed hyperkeratosis with lichenoid inflammation [51]. In 2017, Nguyen et al. reported two cases of oral carcinoma in association with e-cigarette smoking: a 66-year-old who presented with ulceration of the tongue, and a 59-year-old who had an ulcerative lesion on the vermillion of the lower lip. Histopathologic examination in both cases showed basaloid squamous cell carcinoma [52]. In 2021, Klawinski et al. reported a 19-year-old man with a history of vaping using a nicotine-delivery system who presented with a non-healing ulcer on the lateral surface of the tongue. Histopathologic examination revealed a human papillomavirus-negative, poorly differentiated invasive squamous cell carcinoma [53].

Lung Cancer

Lung cancer is the most commonly diagnosed malignant tumor worldwide, with a higher prevalence noted in men compared to women. Based on the International Agency for Research on Cancer, more than 2.5 million new cases of lung cancer are diagnosed globally, mostly in the seventh decade of life [54]. Among its subtypes, small cell lung cancer (SCLC) is the most aggressive, representing about 14% of all lung cancer cases, while adenocarcinoma is the most common histological type, accounting for 38.5% of the cases [55]. While long-term cigarette smoking remains the primary risk factor, the incidence of lung cancer among non-smokers is rising, largely due to air pollution and passive smoking [56]. With the recent surge in e-cigarette use across all age groups worldwide [57, 58], there is growing concern about whether vaping is also a risk factor for lung cancer. A thorough review of the literature shows a lack of unequivocal evidence that e-cigarette use leads to lung cancer. However, as noted at the start of this chapter, numerous studies indicate that e-cigarette chemical compounds and their derivatives following pyrolysis can induce genotoxicity and cellular damage. There is strong evidence suggesting that e-cigarette use incites many of the molecular mechanisms of oncogenesis, including epithelial–mesenchymal transition (EMT), an increase in reactive oxygen species and free radical generation, and DNA damage (breaks and fragmentation) [37, 59, 60]. Tang et al. conducted a study using a murine model and found a significantly higher prevalence of adenocarcinoma in mice exposed to aerosolized e-liquid for 54 weeks compared to those exposed to filtered air (22.5% vs. 5.6%, respectively) [61]. Lee et al. examined the impact of nitrosamines on DNA in mice exposed to e-cigarettes and noted DNA damage, marked reduction in DNA-repair activity, and a significant decrease in repair proteins in the lungs. Moreover, the authors found that nicotine-derived nitrosamine ketone, a metabolite of nicotine, may enhance tumorigenic transformation. The authors concluded that vaping may be carcinogenic to the murine lungs [62]. Using a rat lung model, Canistro et al. found that e-cigarettes can induce DNA damage at chromosomal and gene levels. The authors demonstrated enhancement of phase-1 carcinogen-bioactivating enzymes and a rise in oxygen free radical production. The authors also found an increase in DNA oxidation to 8-hydroxy-2-deoxyguanosine [63]. Hodge et al. reported a decrease in efferocytosis and bacterial phagocytosis following exposure of nontypeable *Haemophilus influenzae* (NTHi) colonies to e-cigarette vapor. Efferocytosis refers to the mechanism of apoptotic cell removal by macrophages and represents the last stage of apoptosis [64]. Using human lung fibroblasts, Lerner et al. demonstrated mitochondria sensitivity to copper nanoparticles in e-cigarette aerosols [65]. Disruption in mitochondrial electron transport and disrupted cellular energetics in turn have been linked to genotoxicity.

Bladder Cancer

Smoking is a well-established cause of bladder cancer, with almost one out of two bladder cancers being caused by tobacco smoke. Various carcinogenic urinary compounds have been identified, including aldehydes, aromatic amines, inorganic compounds, and polyaromatic hydrocarbons [66–69]. Bjurlin et al. stratified urinary biomarkers into two classes: the PAHs and the VOCs. The PAHs are classified as possible or indeterminate carcinogens, whereas VOCs are classified as established carcinogens or indeterminate based on the International Agency for Research on Cancer (IARC) [70, 71]. In a systematic review on carcinogen biomarkers in the urine of e-cigarette users and how they can relate to the development of bladder cancer, Bjurlin et al. showed significant differences in biomarker levels between e-cigarette users and non-tobacco users [70]. It is essential to note that the urine concentrations of these biomarkers, although they are directly related to the frequency and pattern of vaping, also vary among individuals due to differences in metabolic processes and are often confounded or masked by environmental exposures [72–76]. Numerous other studies concurred with the systematic review of Bjurlin et al. Fuller et al. investigated the presence of 5 known bladder carcinogens in 13 e-cigarette users and found 2.3- and 1.3-fold higher concentrations of o-toluidine and 2-naphtylamine, respectively. Nine out of the 13 vapors were long-term non-smokers [77]. Goniewicz et al. measured tobacco-related toxicants in e-cigarette users using urine samples and showed that non-smokers had 19% to 81% lower concentration of biomarkers of exposure to tobacco-specific nitrosamines (TSNAs), volatile organic compounds, and metals such as lead and cadmium. On the other hand, the concentration of many biomarkers was less than that observed in exclusive cigarette smokers. The authors also highlighted the increased concentration of these constituents when both combusted tobacco cigarettes and e-cigarettes are used [74]. Aherrera et al. analyzed nickel (Ni) and chromium (Cr) biomarker levels in e-cigarette users and their association with e-cigarette use patterns in a cohort of 64 vapers using urine, saliva, and exhaled breath condensate. The results showed a median Ni and Cr level of 0.73 and 0.39 microgram/g creatinine in urine. Moreover, an increase in the frequency of vaping was associated with an increase in the Ni biomarker level [78]. Rubinstein investigated the level of chemical toxicants in the saliva and urine of adolescent e-cigarette users. The results showed significantly higher excretion of acrolein, propylene oxide, crotonaldehyde, and acrylamide in comparison to controls. The authors stressed the need to alert e-cigarette users about the carcinogenic potential of these organic compounds [72]. In a study on the oncogenicity of e-cigarette smoke, Tang et al. reported a higher rate of urothelial hyperplasia in FBV/N mice exposed to aerosolized e-liquid, in comparison to those exposed to filtered air [61]. In conclusion, scientific data suggest that e-cigarette compounds, primary or secondary, may cause toxicity and cellular damage, suggesting an increased risk for bladder cancer malignancy.

References

1. Bracken-Clarke D, Kapoor D, Baird AM, Buchanan PJ, Gately K, Cuffe S, Finn SP. Vaping and lung cancer–a review of current data and recommendations. Lung Cancer. 2021;1(153):11–20.
2. de Medeiros KS, Pacheco BF, de Oliveira PE, de Góis Nogueira IL, Diógenes VR, Fernandes FG, Fernandes GC, de Moura Santos E, do Rêgo AC, Araújo-Filho I. Impact of e-cigarettes as cancer risk: a protocol for systematic review and meta-analysis. Medicine. 2023;102(1):e32233
3. Palaia G, Mohsen M, Pergolini D, Bartone V, Purrazzella A, Romeo U, Polimeni A. E-cigarette: a safe tool or a risk factor for oral cancer? A systematic review. J Clin Exp Dent. 2025;17(2):e219.
4. Dela Cruz CS, Tanoue LT, Matthay RA. Lung cancer: epidemiology, etiology, and prevention. Clin Chest Med. 2011;32(4):605–44. https://doi.org/10.1016/j.ccm.2011.09.001. PMID: 22054876; PMCID: PMC3864624
5. Tsai KYF, Hirschi Budge KM, Lepre AP, Rhees MS, Ajdaharian J, Geiler J, Epperson DG, Astle KJ, Winden DR, Arroyo JA, Reynolds PR. Cell invasion, RAGE expression, and inflammation in oral squamous cell carcinoma (OSCC) cells exposed to e-cigarette flavoring. Clin Exp Dent Res. 2020;6(6):618–25. https://doi.org/10.1002/cre2.314. Epub 2020 Aug 11. PMID: 32783323; PMCID: PMC7745078
6. Vermehren MF, Wiesmann N, Deschner J, Brieger J, Al-Nawas B, Kämmerer PW. Comparative analysis of the impact of e-cigarette vapor and cigarette smoke on human gingival fibroblasts. Toxicol In Vitro. 2020;69:105005. https://doi.org/10.1016/j.tiv.2020.105005;. Epub 2020 Sep 18. PMID: 32956835
7. Yu V, Rahimy M, Korrapati A, Xuan Y, Zou AE, Krishnan AR, Tsui T, Aguilera JA, Advani S, Crotty Alexander LE, Brumund KT, Wang-Rodriguez J, Ongkeko WM. Electronic cigarettes induce DNA strand breaks and cell death independently of nicotine in cell lines. Oral Oncol. 2016;52:58–65. https://doi.org/10.1016/j.oraloncology.2015.10.018. Epub 2015 Nov 4. PMID: 26547127; PMCID: PMC4891196.

8. Sancilio S, Gallorini M, Cataldi A, di Giacomo V. Cytotoxicity and apoptosis induction by e-cigarette fluids in human gingival fibroblasts. Clin Oral Investig. 2016;20(3):477–83. https://doi.org/10.1007/s00784-015-1537-x. Epub 2015 Aug 4. PMID: 26239821.
9. de Lima JM, Macedo CCS, Barbosa GV, Castellano LRC, Hier MP, Alaoui-Jamali MA, da Silva SD. E-liquid alters oral epithelial cell function to promote epithelial to mesenchymal transition and invasiveness in preclinical oral squamous cell carcinoma. Sci Rep. 2023;13(1):3330. https://doi.org/10.1038/s41598-023-30016-0. PMID: 36849550; PMCID: PMC9971414
10. Wisniewski DJ, Ma T, Schneider A. Nicotine induces oral dysplastic keratinocyte migration via fatty acid synthase-dependent epidermal growth factor receptor activation. Exp Cell Res. 2018;370(2):343–52. https://doi.org/10.1016/j.yexcr.2018.06.036. Epub 2018 Jun 30. PMID: 29966661; PMCID: PMC6108942.
11. Schwarzmeier LÂT, da Cruz BS, Ferreira CCP, Carvalho BFDC, Alves MGO, Lima Carta CF, Scholz JR, Almeida JD. E-cig might cause cell damage of oral mucosa. Oral Surg Oral Med Oral Pathol Oral Radiol. 2021;131(4):435–43. https://doi.org/10.1016/j.oooo.2020.11.009. Epub 2020 Nov 19. PMID: 33610539.
12. Pandarathodiyil AK, Ramanathan A, Garg R, Doss JG, Abd Rahman FB, Ghani WMN, Warnakulasuriya S. Lactate dehydrogenase levels in the saliva of cigarette and E-cigarette smokers (Vapers): a comparative analysis. Asian Pac J Cancer Prev. 2021;22(10):3227–35. https://doi.org/10.31557/APJCP.2021.22.10.3227. PMID: 34710999; PMCID: PMC8858253
13. Kamal NM, Shams NS. The impact of tobacco smoking and electronic cigarette vaping on salivary biomarkers. A comparative study. Saudi Dent J. 2022;34(5):404–9. https://doi.org/10.1016/j.sdentj.2022.05.003. Epub 2022 May 20. PMID: 35814841; PMCID: PMC9263753
14. Guo J, Hecht SS. DNA damage in human oral cells induced by use of e-cigarettes. Drug Test Anal. 2023;15(10):1189–97. https://doi.org/10.1002/dta.3375. Epub 2022 Oct 4. PMID: 36169810; PMCID: PMC10043052
15. Ye D, Gajendra S, Lawyer G, Jadeja N, Pishey D, Pathagunti S, Lyons J, Veazie P, Watson G, McIntosh S, Rahman I. Inflammatory biomarkers and growth factors in saliva and gingival crevicular fluid of e-cigarette users, cigarette smokers, and dual smokers: a pilot study. J Periodontol. 2020;91(10):1274–83. https://doi.org/10.1002/JPER.19-0457. Epub 2020 Mar 16. PMID: 32052441; PMCID: PMC9014419
16. Hamad SH, Brinkman MC, Tsai YH, Mellouk N, Cross K, Jaspers I, Clark PI, Granville CA. Pilot study to detect genes involved in DNA damage and Cancer in humans: potential biomarkers of exposure to E-cigarette aerosols. Genes (Basel). 2021;12(3):448. https://doi.org/10.3390/genes12030448. PMID: 33809907; PMCID: PMC8004185
17. Kesimer M. Another warning sign: high nicotine content in electronic cigarettes disrupts Muco- ciliary clearance, the essential Defense mechanism of the Lung. Am J Respir Crit Care Med. 2019;200:1082–4.
18. Fahrer J, Christmann M. DNA alkylation damage by nitrosamines and relevant DNA repair pathways. Int J Mol Sci. 2023;24(5):4684. https://doi.org/10.3390/ijms24054684. PMID: 36902118; PMCID: PMC10003415
19. Stepanov I, Carmella SG, Han S, Pinto A, Strasser AA, Lerman C, Hecht SS. Evidence for endogenous formation of N'-nitrosonornicotine in some long-term nicotine patch users. Nicotine Tob Res. 2009;11(1):99–105. https://doi.org/10.1093/ntr/ntn004. Epub 2009 Jan 27. PMID: 19246447; PMCID: PMC2734288.
20. Benowitz NL, Hukkanen J, Jacob P 3rd. Nicotine chemistry, metabolism, kinetics and biomarkers. Handb Exp Pharmacol. 2009;192:29–60. https://doi.org/10.1007/978-3-540-69248-5_2. PMID: 19184645; PMCID: PMC2953858
21. Xue J, Yang S, Seng S. Mechanisms of Cancer induction by tobacco-specific NNK and NNN. Cancers (Basel). 2014;6(2):1138–56. https://doi.org/10.3390/cancers6021138. PMID: 24830349; PMCID: PMC4074821

22. Sahu R, Shah K, Malviya R, Paliwal D, Sagar S, Singh S, Prajapati BG, Bhattacharya S. E-cigarettes and associated health risks: an update on cancer potential. Adv Respir Med. 2023;91(6):516–31.
23. Hakim M, Broza YY, Barash O, Peled N, Phillips M, Amann A, Haick H. Volatile organic compounds of lung cancer and possible biochemical pathways. Chem Rev. 2012;112:5949–66.
24. Cheng T. Chemical evaluation of electronic cigarettes. Tob Control. 2014;23 Suppl 2(Suppl 2):ii11–7. https://doi.org/10.1136/tobaccocontrol-2013-051482. PMID: 24732157; PMCID: PMC3995255
25. Kosmider L, Sobczak A, Fik M, Knysak J, Zaciera M, Kurek J, Goniewicz ML. Carbonyl compounds in electronic cigarette vapors: effects of nicotine solvent and battery output voltage. Nicotine Tob Res. 2014;16:1319–26.
26. Bitzer ZT, Goel R, Reilly SM, Elias RJ, Silakov A, Foulds J, Muscat J, Richie JP Jr. Effect of flavoring chemicals on free radical formation in electronic cigarette aerosols. Free Radic Biol Med. 2018;20(120):72–9. https://doi.org/10.1016/j.freeradbiomed.2018.03.020. Epub 2018 Mar 13. PMID: 29548792; PMCID: PMC5940571
27. Kaur G, Muthumalage T, Rahman I. Mechanisms of toxicity and biomarkers of flavoring and flavor enhancing chemicals in emerging tobacco and non-tobacco products. Toxicol Lett. 2018;15(288):143–55. https://doi.org/10.1016/j.toxlet.2018.02.025. Epub 2018 Feb 23. PMID: 29481849; PMCID: PMC6549714
28. Gerloff J, Sundar IK, Freter R, Sekera ER, Friedman AE, Robinson R, Pagano T, Rahman I. Inflammatory response and barrier dysfunction by different e-cigarette Flavoring chemicals identified by gas chromatography-mass spectrometry in e-liquids and e-Vapors on human Lung epithelial cells and fibroblasts. Appl In Vitro Toxicol. 2017;3(1):28–40. https://doi.org/10.1089/aivt.2016.0030. PMID: 28337465; PMCID: PMC5338075
29. Goniewicz ML, Gawron M, Smith DM, Peng M, Jacob P, III; Benowitzm, N.L. Exposure to nicotine and selected toxicants in cigarette smokers who switched to electronic cigarettes: a longitudinal within-subjects observational study. Nicotine Tob Res. 2017;19:160–7.
30. Brown CJ, Cheng JM. Electronic cigarettes: product characterisation and design considerations. Tob Control. 2014;23:ii4–ii10.
31. Sung H, Ferlay J, Siegel RL, Laversanne M, Soerjomataram I, Jemal A. Global Cancer statistics 2020: GLOBOCAN estimates of incidence and mortality worldwide for 36 cancers in 185 countries. CA Cancer J Clin. 2021;71:209–49.
32. Warnakulasuriya S, Kerr AR. Oral Cancer screening: past, present, and future. J Dent Res. 2021;100:1313–20.
33. Gallagher KP, Vargas PA, Santos-Silva AR. The use of E-cigarettes as a risk factor for oral potentially malignant disorders and oral cancer: a rapid review of clinical evidence. Med Oral Patol Oral Cir Bucal. 2024;29(1):e18–26. https://doi.org/10.4317/medoral.26042. PMID: 37992145; PMCID: PMC10765326
34. Miranda-Filho A, Bray F. Global patterns and trends in cancers of the lip, tongue and mouth. Oral Oncol. 2020;102:104551.
35. Warnakulasuriya S. Oral potentially malignant disorders: a comprehensive review on clinical aspects and management. Oral Oncol. 2020;102:104550.
36. Speight PM, Khurram SA, Kujan O. Oral potentially malignant disorders: risk of progression to malignancy. Oral Surg Oral Med Oral Pathol Oral Radiol. 2018;125:612–27.
37. Abelia XA, Lesmana R, Goenawan H, Abdulah R, Barliana MI. Comparison impact of cigarettes and e-cigs as lung cancer risk inductor: a narrative review. Eur Rev Med Pharmacol Sci. 2023;27(13):6301–18. https://doi.org/10.26355/eurrev_202307_32990. PMID: 37458647
38. Sadri G, Mahjub H. Tobacco smoking and oral cancer: a meta-analysis. Journal of research in health sciences. 2007;7(1):18–23.
39. Zygogianni AG, Kyrgias G, Karakitsos P, Psyrri A, Kouvaris J, Kelekis N, Kouloulias V. Oral squamous cell cancer: early detection and the role of alcohol and smoking. Head Neck Oncol. 2011;6(3):2. https://doi.org/10.1186/1758-3284-3-2. PMID: 21211041; PMCID: PMC3022893

40. Ford PJ, Rich AM. Tobacco use and Oral health. Addiction. 2021;116(12):3531–40. https://doi.org/10.1111/add.15513;. Epub 2021 Apr 25. PMID: 33822437
41. Rom O, Pecorelli A, Valacchi G, Reznick AZ. Are E-cigarettes a safe and good alternative to cigarette smoking? Ann N Y Acad Sci. 2015;1340(1):65–74.
42. Glantz SA, Bareham DW. E-cigarettes: use, effects on smoking, risks, and policy implications. Annu Rev Public Health. 2018;1(39):215–35.
43. Löhler J, Wollenberg B. Are electronic cigarettes a healthier alternative to conventional tobacco smoking? Eur Arch Otorrinolaringol. 2019;276(1):17–25.
44. Bardellini E, Amadori F, Conti G, Majorana A. Oral mucosal lesions in electronic cigarettes consumers versus former smokers. Acta Odontol Scand. 2018;76(3):226–8.
45. Willershausen I, Wolf T, Weyer V, Sader R, Ghanaati S, Willershausen B. Influence of E-smoking liquids on human periodontal ligament fibroblasts. Head Face Med. 2014;10:39.
46. Korrapati A, Yu V, Saad MA, Rahimy M, Xuan Y, Zou A, Krishnan A, Brumund K, Ongkeko WM. The carcinogenic effects of electronic cigarettes in oral cancer. Cancer Res. 2016;76:4069.
47. Bustamante G, Ma B, Yakovlev G, Yershova K, Le C, Jensen J, Hatsukami DK, Stepanov I. Presence of the Carcinogen N'-Nitrosonornicotine in Saliva of E-cigarette Users. Chem Res Toxicol. 2018;31(8):731–8. https://doi.org/10.1021/acs.chemrestox.8b00089. Epub 2018 Jul 30. PMID: 30019582; PMCID: PMC8556657
48. Tommasi S, Caliri AW, Caceres A, Moreno DE, Li M, Chen Y, Siegmund KD, Besaratinia A. Deregulation of biologically significant genes and associated molecular pathways in the Oral epithelium of electronic cigarette users. Int J Mol Sci. 2019;20(3):738. https://doi.org/10.3390/ijms20030738. PMID: 30744164; PMCID: PMC6386888
49. Cheng G, Guo J, Carmella SG, Lindgren B, Ikuemonisan J, Niesen B, Jensen J, Hatsukami DK, Balbo S, Hecht SS. Increased acrolein–DNA adducts in buccal brushings of e-cigarette users. Carcinogenesis. 2022;43(5):437–44.
50. Kamal NM, Shams NS. The impact of tobacco smoking and electronic cigarette vaping on salivary biomarkers. A comparative study. Saudi Dent J. 2022;34(5):404–9.
51. Bartram A, Jones N, Endersby S. Lichenoid eruption associated with use of an e-cigarette. Br J Oral Maxillofac Surg. 2016;54(4):475.
52. Nguyen H, Kitzmiller JP, Nguyen KT, Nguyen C, Bui T. Oral carcinoma associated with chronic use of electronic cigarettes. Otolaryngol. 2017;7:304.
53. Klawinski D, Hanna I, Breslin NK, Katzenstein HM, Indelicato DJ. Vaping the venom: Oral cavity cancer in a young adult with extensive electronic cigarette use. Pediatrics. 2021;147:5.
54. Smolarz B, Łukasiewicz H, Samulak D, Piekarska E, Kołaciński R, Romanowicz H. Lung Cancer-epidemiology, pathogenesis, treatment and molecular aspect (review of literature). Int J Mol Sci. 2025;26(5):2049. https://doi.org/10.3390/ijms26052049. PMID: 40076671; PMCID: PMC11900952
55. Mazouzi C, Kerboua E, Benyahia R, Ferrah N, Aftis R. Lung cancer:"epidemiology and risk factors". Int J Med Phar Drug Re. 2024;8:1.
56. Debieuvre D. Épidémiologie du cancer du poumon: évolution des vingt dernières années [Lung cancer epidemiology: evolution over the last twenty years]. Bull Cancer. 2025;112(3S1):3S3–15. French. https://doi.org/10.1016/S0007-4551(25)00152-3. PMID: 40155074.
57. Soneji SS, Knutzen KE, Villanti AC. Use of flavored e-cigarettes among adolescents, young adults, and older adults: findings from the population assessment for tobacco and health study. Public Health Rep. 2019;134(3):282–92.
58. Thoonen KA, Jongenelis MI. Perceptions of e-cigarettes among Australian adolescents, young adults, and adults. Addict Behav. 2023;1(144):107741.
59. Zhang Y, Sevilla A, Weller R, Wang S, Gitlin MC, Candiotti KA. The role of α7-nicotinic acetylcho- line receptor in a rat model of chronic nicotine-in- duced mechanical hypersensitivity. Neurosci Lett. 2021;743:17.
60. Bozier J, Chivers EK, Chapman DG, Larcombe AN, Bastian NA, Masso-Silva JA, Byun MK, Mc- Donald CF, Crotty Alexander LE, Ween MP. The evolving landscape of e-cigarettes: a Systematic review of recent evidence. Chest. 2020;157:1362–90.

61. Tang MS, Wu XR, Lee HW, Xia Y, Deng FM, Moreira AL, Chen LC, Huang WC, Lepor H. Electronic-cigarette smoke induces lung adenocarcinoma and bladder urothelial hyperplasia in mice. Proc Natl Acad Sci U S A. 2019;116(43):21727–31. https://doi.org/10.1073/pnas.1911321116. Epub 2019 Oct 7. Erratum in: Proc Natl Acad Sci U S A. 2019 Nov 5;116(45):22884. doi: 10.1073/pnas.1918000116; PMID: 31591243; PMCID: PMC6815158
62. Lee HW, Park SH, Weng MW, Wang HT, Huang WC, Lepor H, Wu XR, Chen LC, Tang MS. E-cigarette smoke damages DNA and reduces repair activity in mouse lung, heart, and bladder as well as in human lung and bladder cells. Proc Natl Acad Sci U S A. 2018;115(7):E1560–9. https://doi.org/10.1073/pnas.1718185115. Epub 2018 Jan 29. PMID: 29378943; PMCID: PMC5816191
63. Canistro D, Vivarelli F, Cirillo S, et al. E-cigarettes induce toxicological effects that can raise the cancer risk. Sci Rep. 2017;7(1):2028. https://doi.org/10.1038/s41598017-02317-8. PMID: 28515485; PMCID: PMC5435699
64. Hodge S, Tran HB, Hamon R, Roscioli E, Hodge G, Jersmann H, Ween M, Reynolds PN, Yeung A, Treiberg J, Wilbert S. Nonantibiotic macrolides restore airway macrophage phagocytic function with potential anti-inflammatory effects in chronic lung diseases. Am J Physiol Lung Cell Mol Physiol. 2017;312:L678–87.
65. Lerner CA, Rutagarama P, Ahmad T, Sundar IK, Elder A, Rahman I. Electronic cigarette aerosols and copper nanoparticles induce mitochondrial stress and promote DNA fragmentation in lung fibroblasts. Biochem Biophys Res Commun. 2016;477(4):620–5. https://doi.org/10.1016/j.bbrc.2016.06.109. Epub 2016 Jun 23. PMID: 27343559; PMCID: PMC4967027
66. Riedel K, Scherer G, Engl J, Hagedorn HW, Tricker AR. Determination of three carcinogenic aromatic amines in urine of smokers and nonsmokers. J Anal Toxicol. 2006;30:187–95.
67. Stabbert R, Schäfer KH, Biefel C, Rustemeier K. Analysis of aromatic amines in cigarette smoke. Rapid Commun Mass Spectrom. 2003;17:2125–32.
68. Chen YC, Su HJ, Guo YL, Houseman EA, Christiani DC. Interaction between environmental tobacco smoke and arsenic methylation ability on the risk of bladder cancer. Cancer Causes Control. 2005;16:75–81.
69. Cumberbatch MG, Rota M, Catto JW, La Vecchia C. The role of tobacco smoke in bladder and kidney carcinogenesis: a comparison of exposures and meta-analysis of incidence and mortality risks. Eur Urol. 2015;70:458–66.
70. Bjurlin MA, Matulewicz RS, Roberts TR, Dearing BA, Schatz D, Sherman S, Gordon T, Shahawy OE. Carcinogen biomarkers in the urine of electronic cigarette users and implications for the development of bladder Cancer: a systematic review. Eur Urol Oncol. 2021;4(5):766–83. https://doi.org/10.1016/j.euo.2020.02.004;. Epub 2020 Mar 16. PMID: 32192941
71. Slavin KV, Tesoro EP, Mucksavage JJ. The treatment of cancer pain. Drugs Today (Barc). 2004;40(3):235–45. https://doi.org/10.1358/dot.2004.40.3.820087. PMID: 15148532
72. Rubinstein ML, Delucchi K, Benowitz NL, Ramo DE. Adolescent exposure to toxic volatile organic chemicals from e-cigarettes. Pediatrics. 2018;141(4):e20173557. https://doi.org/10.1542/peds.2017-3557. Epub 2018 Mar 5. PMID: 29507165; PMCID: PMC5869331
73. Shahab L, Goniewicz ML, Blount BC, Brown J, McNeill A, Alwis KU, Feng J, Wang L, West R. Nicotine, carcinogen, and toxin exposure in long-term E-cigarette and nicotine replacement therapy users: a Cross-sectional study. Ann Intern Med. 2017;166(6):390–400. https://doi.org/10.7326/M16-1107. Epub 2017 Feb 7. PMID: 28166548; PMCID: PMC5362067
74. Goniewicz ML, Smith DM, Edwards KC, et al. Comparison of nicotine and toxicant exposure in users of electronic cigarettes and combustible cigarettes. JAMA Netw Open. 2018;1(8):e185937. https://doi.org/10.1001/jamanetworkopen.2018.5937. PMID: 30646298; PMCID: PMC6324349
75. Wagener TL, Floyd EL, Stepanov I, et al. Have combustible cigarettes met their match? The nicotine delivery profiles and harmful constituent exposures of second-generation and third-generation electronic cigarette users. Tob Control. 2017;26(e1):e23–8. https://doi.org/10.1136/tobaccocontrol-2016-053041. Epub 2016 Oct 11. PMID: 27729564; PMCID: PMC5574194.

76. Bekki K, Uchiyama S, Ohta K, Inaba Y, Nakagome H, Kunugita N. Carbonyl compounds generated from electronic cigarettes. Int J Environ Res Public Health. 2014;11(11):11192–200. https://doi.org/10.3390/ijerph111111192. PMID: 25353061; PMCID: PMC4245608
77. Fuller TW, Acharya AP, Meyyappan T, Yu M, Bhaskar G, Little SR, Tarin TV. Comparison of bladder carcinogens in the urine of E-cigarette users versus non E-cigarette using controls. Sci Rep. 2018;8(1):507. https://doi.org/10.1038/s41598-017-19030-1. PMID: 29323232; PMCID: PMC5765148
78. Aherrera A, Olmedo P, Grau-Perez M, Tanda S, Goessler W, Jarmul S, Chen R, Cohen JE, Rule AM, Navas-Acien A. The association of e-cigarette use with exposure to nickel and chromium: a preliminary study of non-invasive biomarkers. Environ Res. 2017;159:313–20. https://doi.org/10.1016/j.envres.2017.08.014;. Epub 2017 Aug 21. PMID: 28837903

Index

A.-l. Hamdan, *E-Cigarette Smoking, Voice, and Health*,
https://doi.org/10.1007/978-3-032-04913-1

GPSR Compliance

The European Union's (EU) General Product Safety Regulation (GPSR) is a set of rules that requires consumer products to be safe and our obligations to ensure this.

If you have any concerns about our products, you can contact us on ProductSafety@springernature.com

In case Publisher is established outside the EU, the EU authorized representative is:

Springer Nature Customer Service Center GmbH
Europaplatz 3
69115 Heidelberg, Germany

Batch number: 09013545

Printed by Printforce, the Netherlands